Psych Meds Made Easy

Callie Parker

Copyright © 2025 by Callie Parker

All rights reserved.

No portion of this book may be reproduced in any form without written permission from the publisher or author, except as permitted by U.S. copyright law.

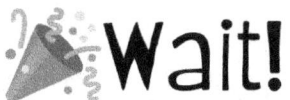 # Wait!

Before You Dive In... Grab Your FREE Nursing Study Survival Kit!

Nursing school is no joke—that's why MadeEasy.Academy is committed to sending the ladder back down and rescuing those of you in the trenches!

Ready to study smarter, not harder? We've got exactly what you need.

Your FREE NCLEX in My Sleep Bundle Includes:

✅ Who's Dying First? The Prioritization Playbook: Because patient safety is kind of a big deal. 😅
✅ Flashcard Frenzy: Memorize or Die Trying: Pre-made Anki cards to save your sanity.
✅ WTF Does This Lab Value Mean? Cheat Sheet: No more second-guessing normal vs. "oh sh*t" levels.
✅ NCLEX Mnemonics That Stick (Like Tape on an IV Line): Memory hacks you'll actually remember.
✅ Med Math Without the Mental Breakdown: Because no one wants to commit a dosage error. 😷

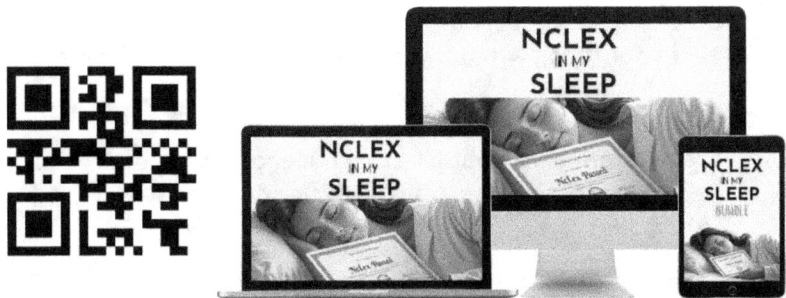

Head over to MadeEasy.Academy to grab your bundle. Let's turn nursing school stress into success!

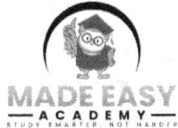

But that's not all...

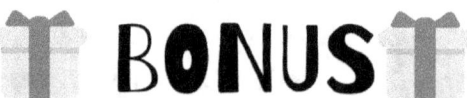

Your Bundle Includes an Exclusive 50% OFF Discount Code for your next course at Made Easy Academy
(Launching June 1!)

At <u>MadeEasy.Academy</u> we don't just simplify nursing—we transform it into an effortless, memorable study process.

For each topic, you'll follow our step by step success guide:

 Step 1. Grab your cheat sheet: All key points, zero fluff.

 Step 2. Read your mnemonic poem: Clever rhymes to make information stick.

 Step 3. Take your fill-in-the-blank quiz: Test your recall without the overwhelm.

 Step 4. Complete your NCLEX challenge: Realistic practice questions with clear rationales.

 Step 5. **Walk Into the NCLEX Like a Boss:** Confident, prepared, and ready to pass.

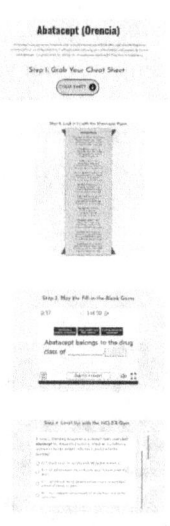
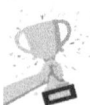

Right now, we're laser-focused on Pharmacology, but we'll soon expand into other crucial nursing topics! Have a topic you want us to cover next? Shoot us an email at hello@madeeasy.academy—we've got you!

Contents

1. Acamprosate (Campral) — 6
2. Alprazolam (Xanax) — 8
3. Amitriptyline (Elavil) — 10
4. Amphetamine/Dextroamphetamine (Adderall, Adderall XR) — 12
5. Aripiprazole (Abilify) — 14
6. Aripiprazole Lauroxil (Aristada) — 16
7. Asenapine (Saphris, Secuado) — 18
8. Atomoxetine (Strattera) — 20
9. Benztropine (Cogentin) — 22
10. Brexpiprazole (Rexulti) — 24
11. Buprenorphine (Subutex, Sublocade) — 26
12. Buprenorphine + Naloxone (Suboxone) — 28
13. Bupropion (Wellbutrin, Zyban) — 30
14. Buspirone (Buspar) — 32
15. Carbamazepine (Tegretol) — 34
16. Cariprazine (Vraylar) — 36
17. Chlordiazepoxide (Librium) — 38
18. Chlorpromazine (Thorazine) — 40
19. Citalopram (Celexa) — 42
20. Clonazepam (Klonopin) — 44

21.	Clonidine (Catapres)	46
22.	Clozapine (Clozaril)	48
23.	Clorazepate (Tranxene)	50
24.	Desvenlafaxine (Pristiq)	52
25.	Desipramine (Norpramin)	54
26.	Dextroamphetamine (Dexedrine, ProCentra, Zenzedi)	56
27.	Dexmethylphenidate (Focalin, Focalin XR)	58
28.	Diazepam (Valium)	60
29.	Diphenhydramine (Benadryl)	62
30.	Disulfiram (Antabuse)	64
31.	Divalproex (Depakote)	66
32.	Doxepin (Silenor, Sinequan)	68
33.	Duloxetine (Cymbalta)	70
34.	Escitalopram (Lexapro)	72
35.	Esketamine (Spravato)	74
36.	Eszopiclone (Lunesta)	76
37.	Flumazenil (Romazicon)	78
38.	Flupentixol (Fluanxol, Depixol)	80
39.	Fluphenazine (Prolixin, Prolixin Decanoate)	82
40.	Fluoxetine (Prozac)	84
41.	Flurazepam (Dalmane)	86
42.	Fluvoxamine (Luvox)	88
43.	Gabapentin (Neurontin)	90
44.	Guanfacine (Intuniv, Tenex)	92
45.	Haloperidol (Haldol)	94
46.	Hydroxyzine (Vistaril, Atarax)	96
47.	Iloperidone (Fanapt)	98
48.	Imipramine (Tofranil)	100

49.	Isocarboxazid (Marplan)	102
50.	Lamotrigine (Lamictal)	104
51.	Lemborexant (Dayvigo)	106
52.	Levomepromazine (Nozinan / Methotrimeprazine)	108
53.	Levomilnacipran (Fetzima)	110
54.	Lisdexamfetamine (Vyvanse)	112
55.	Lithium (Lithobid, Eskalith)	114
56.	Lorazepam (Ativan)	117
57.	Loprazolam (Dormonoct)	119
58.	Lormetazepam (Noctamid)	121
59.	Lumateperone (Caplyta)	123
60.	Lurasidone (Latuda)	125
61.	Melatonin (Circadin, Slenyto, Syncrodin)	127
62.	Memantine (Namenda)	129
63.	Methadone (Dolophine, Methadose)	131
64.	Methylphenidate (Ritalin, Concerta)	133
65.	Midazolam (Versed)	135
66.	Mirtazapine (Remeron)	137
67.	Moclobemide (Aurorix, Manerix)	139
68.	Modafinil (Provigil)	141
69.	Naloxone (Narcan)	143
70.	Naltrexone (ReVia, Vivitrol)	145
71.	Nitrazepam (Mogadon)	147
72.	Nortriptyline (Pamelor)	149
73.	Olanzapine (Zyprexa)	152
74.	Oxazepam (Serax)	154
75.	Oxcarbazepine (Trileptal)	156
76.	Paliperidone (Invega, Invega Sustenna, Invega Trinza)	158

77.	Paroxetine (Paxil)	160
78.	Perphenazine (Trilafon)	163
79.	Phenelzine (Nardil)	165
80.	Pimozide (Orap)	168
81.	Prazosin (Minipress)	170
82.	Propranolol (Inderal)	172
83.	Pregabalin (Lyrica)	175
84.	Protriptyline (Vivactil)	177
85.	Quetiapine (Seroquel)	180
86.	Ramelteon (Rozerem)	183
87.	Risperidone (Risperdal)	185
88.	Selegiline (Eldepryl, Zelapar, Emsam)	187
89.	Serdexmethylphenidate / Dexmethylphenidate (Azstarys)	189
90.	Sertraline (Zoloft)	191
91.	Suvorexant (Belsomra)	193
92.	Temazepam (Restoril)	195
93.	Thiothixene (Navane)	197
94.	Topiramate (Topamax)	199
95.	Tranylcypromine (Parnate)	201
96.	Trazodone (Desyrel)	203
97.	Triazolam (Halcion)	205
98.	Trifluoperazine (Stelazine)	207
99.	Trimipramine (Surmontil)	209
100.	Valproate (Depakote, Depakene, Valproic Acid)	211
101.	Venlafaxine (Effexor, Effexor XR)	213
102.	Vilazodone (Viibryd)	215
103.	Vortioxetine (Trintellix)	217
104.	Zaleplon (Sonata)	219

105.	Ziprasidone (Geodon)	221
106.	Zolpidem (Ambien)	223

WHY Made Easy Works

Backed by Brain Science

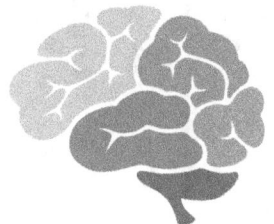

Let's face it — nursing school can feel like trying to drink from a firehose. Between the jargon, the never-ending lists, and the sheer volume of information, it's easy to feel overwhelmed. That's exactly why the Made Easy series was born: to make the hard stuff stick without frying your brain. And while it might look fun and playful on the outside (hello, rhymes!), it's all built on rock-solid research from the nerdy world of educational psychology.

1. COGNITIVE LOAD THEORY

First up: Cognitive Load Theory. Fancy name, simple idea — your brain can only handle so much at once. When materials are too dense or packed with fluff, your working memory taps out. Educational psychologist John Sweller figured this out, and we took notes. That's why our poems give you the essentials only, in small, memorable doses. Less clutter, more clarity. (Sweller, 1988; Clark et al., 2006)

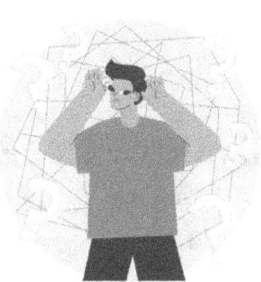

2. DUAL CODING THEORY

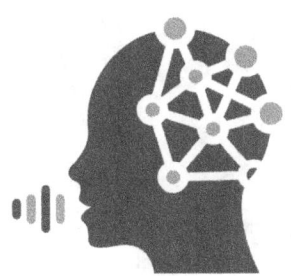

Then there's Dual Coding Theory, brought to us by Allan Paivio. He discovered that we remember things better when we learn them through both words and visuals. Our poems lean into this by using rhyme and rhythm to boost verbal memory — and bolded key terms, color coding, and clean formatting to give your visual brain a treat. Two paths to your brain = double the retention. (Paivio, 1986; Mayer, 2009)

3. ADVANCE ORGANIZERS

Psychologist David Ausubel believed that when we know how new info fits into what we already know, we learn faster. That's the beauty of our repeatable poem structure. Once you get the hang of the format, your brain relaxes — and focuses on what actually matters: the content. Think of it like a familiar playlist for your mind. (Ausubel, 1960)

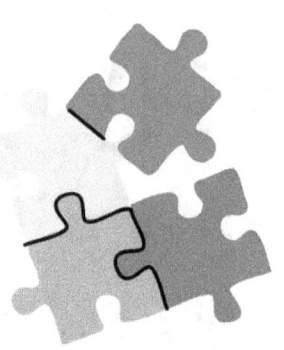

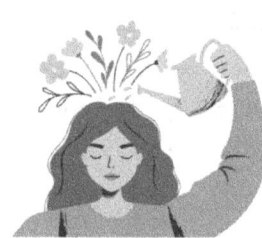

4. MICROLEARNING

Our poems are also bite-sized by design, and that's no accident. Welcome to the world of microlearning — the idea that small, focused learning units are easier to digest and retain. This is a game-changer for busy, burnt-out students. Instead of cramming for hours, you can study just one medication, one skill, or one critical concept at a time. Snack-sized studying with full-course impact. (Hug, 2005; van den Berg & van den Berg, 2021)

5. SPACED REPETITION & RETRIEVAL PRACTICE

Last but definitely not least: spaced repetition and retrieval practice. These two learning powerhouses have proven time and again that the more often you recall information over time, the longer you'll remember it. Our poems are made for this. Easy to reread, perfect for flashcards, and fun enough to come back to (yes, we admitted it). Rinse and repeat — and retain. (Dunlosky et al., 2013)

So, yes — this method might look different than your typical textbook grind. That's the point. It's effective on purpose. Because learning tough topics shouldn't feel impossible. It should feel doable. Even a little fun. And with Made Easy, it totally is.

Read it. Rhyme it. Remember it.

That's the Made Easy Method—a simple but powerful approach to mastering complex nursing material.

ONE — THIS ISN'T REGULAR POETRY—IT'S PURPOSEFUL

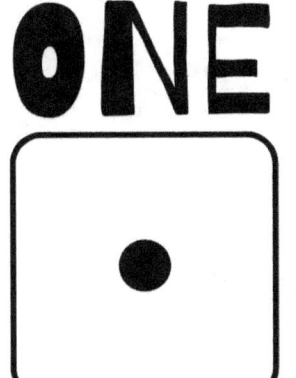

These poems weren't made to be skimmed or read once.
They're built for memory. They're built for you.

They might feel dense at first. You might pause. That's okay.
You're supposed to wrestle with the words.
It's in that wrestling—the rereading, the out-loud reciting, the highlighting—that retention starts to kick in.

Let the rhythm do the heavy lifting.
Rhyme and repetition are memory's best friends.
This poetry is built for practice, not perfection.

TWO — COLOR-CODE FOR CLARITY

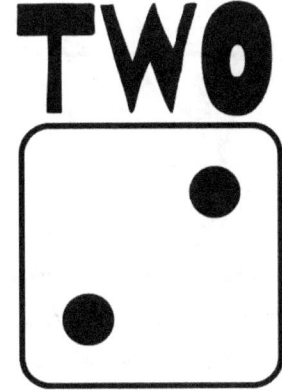

To help you organize and absorb the content, we recommend using a color-coded system while you read.

Highlight or mark up key details with consistent colors for:

- 🟦 Drug Classification & Names
- 🟦 Mechanism of Action
- 🟦 Indications
- 🟦 Side Effects & Adverse Reactions
- 🟦 Nursing Considerations
- ☐ Monitoring Requirements
- 🟦 Patient & Caregiver Teaching Points
- ⬤ Black Box Warnings
- 🟦 Pediatric Considerations
- ⬤ Drug Interactions

When you revisit the poem, your highlights will guide your recall and make review sessions faster and easier.

THREE

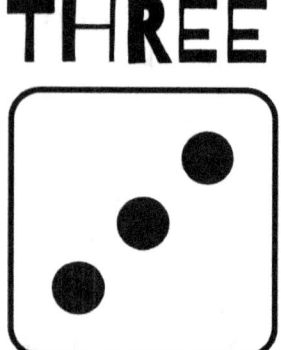

TEST WHAT YOU KNOW

After each section, you'll find a QR code that takes you straight to a short NCLEX-style quiz hosted in Google Forms. These aren't just random practice questions — they're carefully crafted to test the most important takeaways from what you just read. But the real magic? <u>The rationales.</u> Whether you get the answer right or wrong, the quiz walks you through the why. Understanding the reasoning behind each answer helps you think like a nurse, not just a test-taker.

It's not about memorizing — it's about making connections, strengthening critical thinking, and applying your knowledge in real clinical scenarios. So take your time, review the rationales, and let them guide you from confusion to clarity.

So don't just read these pages—
interact with them.

📖 **Read** it.

🎵 **Rhyme** it.

🧠 **Remember** it.

That's how we make nursing Made Easy.

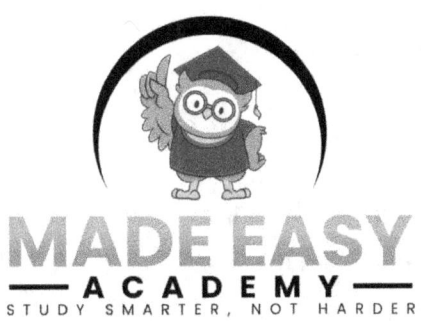

Acamprosate (Campral)

GABA Agonist / Glutamate Modulator – Alcohol Use Disorder Treatment

Acamprosate, recovery's friend,
Helps when alcohol comes to an end.
Supports the brain in **newfound peace**,
By calming the **cravings** that never cease.
Used for **alcohol use disorder** strong,
To keep folks **sober** and going long.
It **restores neurotransmitter flow**,
GABA up, **glutamate** down low.

It doesn't help with **withdrawal pain**,
But helps **prevent relapse** from the strain.
Only works when drinking's stopped—
So don't start it while shots are popped.
Oral tablets, three times daily,
With or without food—it's taken stably.
Renal dosing is a **must-do** step—
If **CrCl is low**, you gotta prep.

Side effects? They're mostly light:

Diarrhea leads, **gas**, and sleep at night.

Sometimes **anxiety**, or **headache**, too,

But nothing major for most to chew.

No Black Box Warning, but nurse, take note:

It's not for use in those **renal bloat**.

CrCl <30? You'll hold that med—

And monitor mood while pushing ahead.

Teach: It won't **stop withdrawal's spin**,

But helps once **detox** work begins.

Not addictive, no liver pain,

Unlike some meds in this same lane.

Acamprosate, a steady guide,

To help the **sober brain** re-align inside.

With nurse support and honest pace,

You'll help them hold their healing space.

Alprazolam (Xanax)

Benzodiazepine – Anxiolytic / CNS Depressant

Alprazolam, the calm in a storm,
A **benzo** that helps the nerves conform.
Used for **panic**, **anxiety's wave**,
It tames the mind so folks feel brave.
It boosts **GABA**, that chill brain brake,
Slows the **CNS** for calm's own sake.
Fast-acting, short-half life delight,
But habit-forming if used too tight.

Oral tabs, and **ODTs** too,
TID or PRN—depends on who.
Watch for **tolerance**, **dependence**, climb,
This ain't a med for all-the-time.
Side effects? They roll in fast:
Drowsy, **dizzy**, memory won't last.
Depression, **confusion**, **falls** in age,
And **CNS depression** takes the stage.

Black Box Warning in bold,
For **benzo + opioid** danger told

Respiratory arrest can strike on cue,
So **no mixing** unless the doc tells you.
Withdrawals hit hard if stopped too quick—
Think **seizures, insomnia, panic kick**.
So **taper slowly**, always nurse-led,
Don't let abrupt stops mess the head.

Not for **pregnancy**—category D,
Cleft palate risk? Potentially.
And if the patient has **substance past**,
This drug's risk climbs up real fast.
Teach: Take it **only as prescribed**,
And **not with booze** or you'll feel fried.
Avoid driving, work machines,
And check in if the mood careens.

Alprazolam—quick calm in hand,
But needs a **nurse who understands**.
With structure, care, and patient trust,
You'll guide this med with focus and just.

Amitriptyline (Elavil)

Tricyclic Antidepressant (TCA) – Mood Stabilizer / Neuropathic Pain Agent

Amitriptyline, old-school med,
Lifts the lows inside your head.
A **TCA**, it blocks the gate
Of **serotonin** and **norepinephrine's** fate.
Used for **depression**, dark and deep,
And **chronic pain** that doesn't sleep.
Also helps with **migraine's fire**,
Or **insomnia** when nerves are wired.

But yo—this med don't play around,
Its **side effect** list is profound.
It's **anticholinergic** to the bone—
Think **dry mouth**, **blurred vision**, leave it alone.
Constipation, urinary hold,
Sedation heavy, stories told.
And weight gain, mood swings, funky dreams,
Are part of this med's vintage themes.

Black Box Warning loud and clear:

Suicidal thoughts in youth appear.

So monitor **mood**, and energy spikes,

Especially in **teens** and younger tykes.

Wanna know what's worst of all?

Amitriptyline's **lethal in overdose call**.

Cardiotoxic, QT prolongs—

A few too many, and it's gone wrong.

EKG before you go all in,

Especially if there's heart history within.

Hold in **MI, seizure crew**,

And use with caution in the **elderly**, too.

Teach: Take it at **night**, it's sedating,

And don't stop fast—**taper** the waiting.

No alcohol, no sleepy pills,

And rise up slow to avoid the chills.

Amitriptyline—retro fire,

With benefits and risks that require

A nurse with **judgment**, eyes on alert,

To give this med without the hurt.

Amphetamine/Dextroamphetamine (Adderall, Adderall XR)

CNS Stimulant – ADHD / Narcolepsy Agent

Adderall, focus in a tab,
A **CNS stimulant** that works real fab.
Mix of **amphetamine** and its twin,
It kicks the **dopamine** drive within.
Used for **ADHD** minds that race,
To help them **slow**, **prioritize**, and **pace**.
Also treats **narcolepsy's sleep**,
So folks don't crash when life runs deep.

It boosts both **norepinephrine** and **dopamine**,
To help that **frontal lobe** realign.
Improves **attention**, **task control**,
But comes with rules to keep it whole.
Oral tabs or **XR caps** each day,
Often first thing—**morning play**.
Watch out if taken **late at night**,
It may disrupt that **sleepy flight**.

Side effects? They're stimulant loud:
Insomnia, **weight loss**, head in a cloud.
Dry mouth, **tics**, or mood that dips,
And **tachycardia** with racing flips.
Black Box Warning stands up tall:
Risk of **abuse** and **dependency** call.
So monitor closely, watch the signs—
Especially in folks with **addictive lines**.

Contra in **cardiac disease**,
Or **HTN** that won't appease.
Also avoid in **anxiety crew**,
Or **bipolar**—mania might break through.
Teach: Take it **whole**, don't crush the shell,
And store it safe (yeah, lock it well).
Monitor height and weight in youth,
And check for **behavioral shifts** in truth.

Adderall—the dopamine drive,
That helps the busy brain **arrive**.
But needs a nurse with structured plan,
To keep it safe in every hand.

Aripiprazole (Abilify)

Atypical Antipsychotic – Dopamine Stabilizer / Mood Agent

Aripiprazole, Abilify fame,
Plays a **dopamine-modulating game**.
It's not just blocking all the way—
It's a **partial agonist** in play.
Used for **schizophrenia's voice**,
Or **bipolar mania's racing choice**.
Also treats **MDD adjunct-style**,
And **autism-related** mood compile.

Helps with **irritability, mood swings wide**,
Brings **stability** to what's inside.
Oral tablets, **ODTs**, or **shots** that stay—
The **long-acting injection** lasts 30-day.
Side effects? They're usually mild,
But still can hit the **sensitive child**.
Akathisia, that inner twitch,
Restlessness that makes folks itch.

Also **weight gain**, though less than peers,
And **insomnia** in some volunteers.

Watch for **EPS**, though risk is low,
Like **dystonia** or a slowed-down flow.
Black Box Warning, double check:
Suicidal thoughts in youth, what the heck.
Also in **dementia psychosis**, beware—
Increased **death risk** hangs out there.

May raise **blood sugar**, **cholesterol**, too,
So monitor labs as nurses do.
Also may increase **impulse behaviors**—
Like **gambling**, **bingeing**, mood-like wavers.
Teach: Take it **daily**, same time style,
Effects may take a **couple weeks' mile**.
Don't stop fast—**taper slow**,
Or relapse symptoms might just grow.

Aripiprazole, flexible friend,
But needs close watching to safely blend.
With **labs**, **teaching**, and structure tight,
You'll guide this med from wrong to right.

Aripiprazole Lauroxil (Aristada)

Atypical Antipsychotic – Long-Acting Injectable (LAI)

Aripiprazole Lauroxil, long and strong,
Keeps the **psychosis** from drifting wrong.
It's **Abilify's cousin**, slow to shine,
Built to **release over weeks of time**.
Used for **schizophrenia's chronic care**,
To help with **relapse prevention** there.
It keeps **dopamine** in check and play,
With a **partial agonist** kind of way.

It's given **IM**, not every day—
Just **once monthly**, or longer delay.
441 to 1064 mg,
Every **4 to 8 weeks**, depending on plan.
But wait—before this shot goes in,
Start with **oral overlap** to win.
You'll need **oral aripiprazole** ride
For **21 days** while LAI's inside.

Side effects? They may arise:
Akathisia, that restless guise.

Sedation, **weight gain**, **anxiety**, too,
Though less than other SGA crew.
Black Box Warning—take it in stride:
In **elderly dementia**, don't let it slide.
Risk of **death** is raised in that space,
So **off-label use** is out of place.

Watch for **neuroleptic malignant syndrome**,
With **fever**, **rigidity**, symptoms that come.
Also monitor for **impulse control**,
Like **gambling** urges that take a toll.
Labs? Watch **lipids**, **glucose**, **weight**,
And **injection site**—keep it great.
Teach that this is **not a cure**,
But part of staying **safe and secure**.

Aristada, slow and smooth,
A long-term antipsychotic groove.
With **nurse-led care** and structured guide,
You'll help your patients **stabilize** with pride.

Asenapine (Saphris, Secuado)

Atypical Antipsychotic – Dopamine & Serotonin Receptor Antagonist

Asenapine, subtle and slick,
Works on **dopamine** fast and quick.
An **SGA** that blocks the storm,
In **mood and thought**, it brings reform.
Used for **schizophrenia's broken track**,
And **bipolar mania's** racing back.
Also used for **mixed mood states**,
To calm the storm before it escalates.

Comes in a **sublingual tab**, not to chew,
It **melts under the tongue**—yeah, that's your clue.
Also a **patch** (Secuado's name),
For those who can't do pills the same.
Side effects? Let's talk them through:
Somnolence, weight gain, and **akathisia**, too.
Oral numbness from sublingual use,
And **orthostatic drops** that cut loose.

Black Box Warning, like most SGA:

Dementia psychosis? Keep away.

Risk of **stroke** and **death** is real,

So this off-label path's a no-deal deal.

Watch for **NMS**, rare but bold,

Muscle stiff, fever, symptoms cold.

Check for **impulse control** gone wild,

Like gambling where it's uncompiled.

Teach: **No food or drink for 10 mins** post-dose,

Or **absorption drops**—you miss the most.

And if using the **patch**, place with care,

Rotate sites, and don't stick on hair.

Asenapine, the stealthy star,

Delivers calm without going far.

With **nurse-led checks** and structure tight,

You'll guide this med with patient insight.

Atomoxetine (Strattera)

Selective Norepinephrine Reuptake Inhibitor (NRI) – Non-Stimulant ADHD Agent

Atomoxetine, focus slow,

Not a stim, but helps brains grow.

It boosts the **norepinephrine track**,

To bring that **attention** and **impulse** back.

Used for **ADHD** in both **young and old**,

But works best when **habits hold**.

Not a med for **quick fix pain**,

It builds up slowly in the brain.

Oral dosing, once or split,

Takes a few **weeks** for full benefit.

Start it low, then titrate right,

Until the focus comes to light.

Side effects? Let's run the list:

Dry mouth, nausea, dizzy twist.

Decreased appetite, mood shifts, too—

And possible **GI issues** may come through.

Black Box Warning, hear it loud:

Suicidal thoughts in the young crowd.

So monitor **mood** and **energy** turns,

Especially in teens—where emotion burns.

Also may **raise BP and pulse**,

So vitals checks are never false.

Not for patients with **liver strain**,

Or **cardiac issues** in the lane.

No abuse potential, no Schedule stamp,

But it still needs care—not a campus champ.

Don't stop fast—taper slow,

And **monitor weight and height** as they grow.

Teach: Take it **same time every day**,

And let it build in a steady way.

Don't expect an **instant shift**,

This med is more of a long-term lift.

Atomoxetine, focus fuel,

Non-stim choice with a different rule.

With nurse support and patient grace,

You'll guide this med in every case.

Benztropine (Cogentin)

Anticholinergic – Parkinson's & EPS Treatment

Benztropine, smooths the scene,
Anticholinergic, crisp and clean.
Used in **Parkinson's tremor ride**,
Or when **antipsychotics** hit too wide.
Treats **EPS** like **dystonia tight**,
And **akathisia**—restless night.
Helps with **rigidity**, muscle sway,
When dopamine's been stripped away.

It blocks **acetylcholine's** loud call,
To bring **motor balance** back overall.
A balance med, not dopamine true—
But makes the movement smoother for you.
Oral or IM, it's PRN style,
Often used for **acute EPS trial**.
But sometimes given as **scheduled care**,
In **Parkinson's** folks who need it there.

Side effects? Oh you know the song:
Dry mouth, **blurred vision**, bowels gone wrong.

Urinary retention, **confusion**, risk—
Especially in **older**—they feel the twist.
No Black Box Warning, but nurse beware:
It's **anticholinergic everywhere**.
Avoid in **glaucoma**, **BPH**, and heat—
It can block sweat, which isn't sweet.

Teach: **Rise up slow**, orthostatic game,
And watch for **memory gaps** or **name**.
Hydrate well, chew gum if dry,
And don't mix with meds that also try.
Monitor for **toxic psychosis** signs,
Especially when dose climbs or aligns.
And know it won't fix the cause inside—
Just helps when symptoms coincide.

Benztropine, the quiet shield,
That guards when movement gets unsealed.
With **nurse precision**, timing tight,
You'll give this med just right each night.

Brexpiprazole (Rexulti)

Atypical Antipsychotic – Dopamine & Serotonin Partial Agonist

Brexpiprazole, mood's soft tune,
Brings **dopamine balance** to the room.
It's not a blocker all the way—
A **partial agonist**, like they say.
Used in **schizophrenia**, calm the mind,
And **adjunct in MDD**, re-aligned.
When **SSRIs** can't lift the shade,
Rexulti helps that progress made.

It modulates **5HT1A, D2**,
For **mood**, **thought**, and **clarity** too.
Less risk of **EPS distress**,
But still needs nurse to **monitor best**.
Oral tablets, once per day,
Start at **low dose**, work your way.
Half-life's long, so steady rise—
Takes **1-4 weeks** to stabilize.

Side effects to track and name:

Akathisia is still fair game.

Also **weight gain, insomnia, GI flow,**

And **agitation** may sometimes show.

Black Box Warning stands its ground:

Suicidal thoughts in youth are found.

Also in **elderly dementia's** lane,

Increased risk of **stroke and pain**.

Teach: Take it **daily**, don't skip the ride,

Even if they start to feel alright inside.

No **sudden stop**—that's not the move,

Let the provider slowly remove.

Monitor **mood, metabolic scale,**

A1C, lipids, weight detail.

And assess for **gambling, compulsions**, flare—

Rare, but possible, so be aware.

Brexpiprazole, a gentle guide,

For thoughts and moods that crash and slide.

With **nurse support** and structured care,

You'll help them stabilize and repair.

Buprenorphine (Subutex, Sublocade)

Partial Opioid Agonist – Opioid Use Disorder Treatment / Pain Management

Buprenorphine, steady and bold,
Helps when **opioid cravings** take hold.
A **partial mu-opioid agonist** true,
It tames withdrawal, but won't get you through.
Used for **opioid use disorder** first,
It **blocks the high**, but calms the worst.
Also used in **chronic pain**,
With **ceiling effect** to curb the strain.

Sublingual tabs or **monthly shot**,
Sublocade lasts a steady slot.
Start it **after withdrawal's begun**,
Too early? **Precip withdrawal** will run.
Side effects? Let's break that down:
Constipation, sedation, dizzy town.
Sweating, headache, nausea, too—
Though milder than full opioids do.

BUPRENORPHINE (SUBUTEX, SUBLOCADE)

Black Box Warning stands in light:

Respiratory depression, **abuse** in sight.

Especially if mixed with **benzos** or **booze**,

It's sedation city—you could lose.

Not for folks with **severe liver strain**,

So monitor **LFTs** to explain.

Watch for **QT prolongation**, rare,

So an **EKG** might be fair.

Teach: **No cutting, chewing, crush or mix**,

It's **sublingual only**, not quick fix.

And when on **Sublocade monthly dose**,

They need to know it **stays in close**.

No driving till they know their feel,

And **lock it up**—this med is real.

CURES or **PDMP** may be in use,

To track the fills and avoid abuse.

Buprenorphine, hope in form,

Keeps recovery steady and warm.

With **nurse support**, **no judgment zone**,

You'll help them rebuild—stone by stone.

Buprenorphine + Naloxone (Suboxone)

Partial Opioid Agonist + Opioid Antagonist – OUD Maintenance Treatment

Suboxone, the gold-standard blend,
For when the spiral needs to end.
Buprenorphine, partial calm,
Eases pain and cravings' qualm.
But then there's **Naloxone** in the ride,
To block abuse if misapplied.
It's **inactive under the tongue**, no lie—
But if **injected**, it makes you **withdraw and cry**.

Used for **opioid use disorder**, straight,
It helps **prevent relapse** at the gate.
It **blocks the high**, yet holds withdrawal,
A **maintenance med** for a stable call.
Given **sublingual**—strip or tab,
Once daily, with a steady grab.
Start it only **after withdrawal shows**,
Or **precipitated hell** explodes.

Side effects? Let's keep it tight:
Headache, sweating, sleepy night.
Constipation, dizzy, mouth goes dry,
But safer than opioids—no lie.
Black Box Warning applies still:
Respiratory depression with the wrong pill.
Especially when **benzos, booze,** or more
Are **mixed together**—hit the floor.

Monitor for **hepatotoxic risk,**
And avoid with liver **labs gone brisk.**
Not for **pain,** not for fun,
This med is serious, not just one-and-done.
Teach: **No cutting, chewing, or gulp,**
Place **under the tongue**—not like a pulp.
No **eating or drinking** till it's clear,
Or the **bioavailability disappears.**

Suboxone—judgment-free care,
For people fighting to repair.
With **structure, support,** and **nursing grace,**
You'll help them heal and find their place.

Bupropion (Wellbutrin, Zyban)

Atypical Antidepressant – NDRI / Smoking Cessation Aid

Bupropion, the uplift spark,
For **depression** stuck in the dark.
It boosts both **dopamine** and **NE**,
But skips the **serotonin** recipe.
Called a **NDRI** by name,
It fights the fog without the flame.
Used for **MDD** and **seasonal blues**,
And **smoking cessation** (that's Zyban's use).

Off-label ADHD? Yup, it's there,
For patients needing dopamine care.
Comes in **IR**, **SR**, and **XL** form,
Dosed based on what's to transform.
Side effects? Let's name a few:
Insomnia, **dry mouth**, nervous too.
Weight loss often comes along,
No **sexual side effects**? That's strong.

Black Box Warning, just like the rest:
Suicidal thoughts in the youthful test.

And the **seizure threshold**—very low,

Especially when **doses go** too slow or grow.

Also contraindicated if:

They've got **seizure disorder**, or **ED hx**.

Also avoid in **anorexia**,

Or **alcohol withdrawal**, with extra care-ia.

Teach: **Don't double up** if you miss a beat,

Spacing doses is key to keep.

Take **in the morning**, avoid sleep hit,

Unless it's SR—then **split the bit**.

No **abuse potential**, no sedative trend,

But gives that **energizing blend**.

With careful use and nursing flow,

This med can really help them grow.

Bupropion—dopamine drive,

Helps them think, feel, and come alive.

With nurse support and insight clear,

You'll guide this med with bold, calm cheer.

Buspirone (Buspar)

Anxiolytic – Serotonin Partial Agonist (5-HT1A)

Buspirone, the slow and steady,
An **anxiety med** that keeps you ready.
No sedation, no withdrawal fear,
Just takes a while to persevere.
It binds to **5-HT1A**,
Modulates **serotonin's sway**.
Dopamine tweaks? A little touch,
But not enough to make it much.

Used for **GAD**—that chronic dread,
Not for panic's lightning spread.
It **won't sedate**, and **won't depress**,
It's not a fix for acute distress.
Oral tabs, divided dose,
Two to three times daily—close.
Takes about **2-4 weeks to rise**,
Before relief will stabilize.

Side effects are mild at best:
Dizziness, headache, GI unrest.

No weight gain or sleepy cloud,
That's why some folks say it's allowed.
No Black Box Warning, but caution wins:
No MAOIs—can't be twins.
Risk of **hypertensive crisis** there,
So space **14 days** with care.

Teach: Take it **same time every day**,
And don't expect a magic spray.
Not a "take-as-needed" friend—
It's **maintenance dosing** to the end.
No **abuse**, no **addiction game**,
No **controlled substance** in its name.
That's why it's loved for those who fear
Benzo risks that draw too near.

Buspirone—slow calm in view,
No high, no crash, just pushing through.
With nurse-led timing, teaching clear,
You'll guide this med through every fear.

Carbamazepine (Tegretol)

Anticonvulsant / Mood Stabilizer – Sodium Channel Blocker

Carbamazepine, strong and clean,
A **sodium blocker** in the neural scene.
Used for **bipolar, seizures, nerve pain**,
It keeps the highs and shocks in lane.
Mania moods? It chills the tide.
Trigeminal neuralgia? Cuts pain's ride.
Also used for **partial seizures** tight—
But needs some labs to guide it right.

Oral tabs, extended too,
Take with **food** so nausea's through.
Therapeutic range is key to show:
Aim for **4 to 12 mcg/mL flow**.
Side effects you need to know:
Drowsiness, dizzy, ataxia show.
Nausea, blurred vision, rash, and more,
So start it slow and monitor.

Black Box Warnings, heavy and loud:
Aplastic anemia in the crowd.

And serious **agranulocytosis**,

So watch those **WBCs** with focus.

Another : In **Asian descent**,

Check for **HLA-B*1502** percent.

Risk of **Stevens-Johnson syndrome** rises,

So test before the dose surprises.

Also induces **CYP450**,

So many drug levels may dip low.

It lowers **oral contraceptives**, too—

So teach what backup plans to do.

Teach: No **grapefruit juice** with this med,

And **don't stop suddenly**, or seizures spread.

Take **same time daily**, and monitor signs

Of **infection**, **bruising**, or **mood declines**.

Carbamazepine—strong, intense,

But brings the brain some calm defense.

With **labs**, **teaching**, and nursing sight,

You'll keep this mood med running right.

Cariprazine (Vraylar)

Atypical Antipsychotic – Dopamine D2/D3 Partial Agonist

Cariprazine, fresh on scene,
Targets **dopamine D3** like a dream.
Used for **schizophrenia's thought dismay**,
And **bipolar**—depressed or manic sway.
Also paired with **SSRIs**,
For **MDD** that lingers and hides.
It **modulates dopamine**, not blocks it cold,
With **partial agonist** control that's bold.

It hits **D2** and **D3** both in line,
But that **D3 preference**? By design.
Helps with **motivation**, **drive**, and flow,
Where **flat affect** and apathy grow.
Oral dosing, once a day,
Long **half-life** means it likes to stay.
Start **low and slow**, and go with grace,
Takes **weeks to reach a steady state** pace.

Side effects? Let's break the trend:
Akathisia is common, my friend.

Also **insomnia**, **nausea**, and a rise
In **restlessness** behind the eyes.
Black Box Warning loud and clear:
Suicidal thoughts in youth appear.
And in **dementia psychosis** land,
There's risk of **death**—don't let it stand.

Lower risk for **weight gain wild**,
Compared to others, it's more mild.
But monitor still for **lipids** and **sugar**,
Because **metabolic shifts** can still occur.
Teach: It takes time to **feel the lift**,
This isn't a quick or sudden shift.
No abrupt stop, and watch for signs
Of **mood swings**, **gambling**, or **compulsive lines**.

Cariprazine, the subtle spark,
That lights the brain when it feels dark.
With **nurse-led checks** and long-term plan,
You'll help this med do all it can.

Chlordiazepoxide (Librium)

Benzodiazepine – Anxiolytic / Alcohol Withdrawal Agent

Chlordiazepoxide, benzo prime,
First on the scene in calming time.
Used for **anxiety**, **tension's blast**,
And **alcohol withdrawal** coming fast.
It **potentiates GABA** in the brain,
Slows the signals, numbs the strain.
Reduces **seizure** risk in detox fight,
While keeping **agitation** out of sight.

Given **oral**—caps or tab,
Long **half-life** means steady grab.
Takes the edge off **tremors**, **sweats**,
And **hallucinations** the brain forgets.
Side effects? Let's lay 'em out:
Drowsiness, **dizzy**, slurred mouth route.
Ataxia, confusion in older crew,
And long-term use brings **tolerance** too.

Black Box Warning lights the way:
Respiratory depression if you play

With **opioids**, alcohol, sleepy meds—
That combo risk can leave folks dead.
Also risk for **dependence high**,
So use it short-term—don't let it lie.
Taper slow if it's time to stop,
Or **withdrawal** could make symptoms pop.

Teach: No **driving**, **alcohol**, or heavy lifts,
And watch for **mood or behavior shifts**.
Take it **as prescribed**, don't break the dose,
And **lock it up**—that's diagnosis-close.
Chlordiazepoxide, Librium's name,
An old-school chill with detox fame.
With **nurse-led care**, structure tight,
You'll guide this med both day and night.

Chlorpromazine (Thorazine)

Typical Antipsychotic – First-Generation / Phenothiazine Class

Chlorpromazine, first in line,
Made psychosis **sedate** and **decline**.
It blocks **dopamine D2** on cue,
To calm **hallucinations** and **delusions**, too.
Used for **schizophrenia's psychotic break**,
And **manic agitation's** mental quake.
Also helps with **nausea**, **hiccups**, weird,
And **intractable vomiting** when it's feared.
IM, **oral**, or **IV** stream,
In **psych units**, it's a common theme.
Starts low, go slow, watch the feel—
This med hits hard, old-school real.
Side effects? Now brace the list:
Sedation, dry mouth, can't resist.
Orthostatic hypotension, blurred sight,
And **photosensitivity** in sunlight.

But here come the **EPS signs**:
Dystonia, akathisia lines.

CHLORPROMAZINE (THORAZINE)

Parkinsonism shuffle step,

And **tardive dyskinesia** if it's kept.

Black Box Warning on the page:

Not for **elderly psychosis age**.

In **dementia patients**, risk is real—

Higher chance they won't heal.

Can trigger **neuroleptic malignant storm**—

High fever, **rigid**, way off norm.

So watch for **NMS**, labs, and tone,

And **hold the med** if that's shown.

Anticholinergic effects come, too:

Constipation, **retention**, drying through.

So push fluids, walk, and teach

To avoid the symptoms that overreach.

Teach: Avoid the sun, **rise up slow**,

No alcohol—let that go.

Take **with food** if GI's mad,

And **report any twitch** or feelin' bad.

Chlorpromazine—Thorazine style,

Old but powerful, still on file.

With **nurse-led checks** and psych team pride,

You'll keep this med on the safest side.

Citalopram (Celexa)

SSRI – Selective Serotonin Reuptake Inhibitor

Citalopram, a serotonin lift,
For **depression's fog** and mental drift.
It blocks the reuptake **nice and slow**,
To help those mood waves start to flow.
Used for **MDD** and **anxious minds**,
Though not for panic most of the time.
It's often first in **SSRI class**,
For patients needing a gentler pass.
Oral med, take **once per day**,
Usually **morning** to start the way.
Start low, go slow, and let them know—
It takes **2-4 weeks** before it'll show.
Side effects? Let's make it clear:
Nausea, dry mouth, maybe **sleepy gear**.
Sexual dysfunction often seen,
And **weight changes** sneak between.

Black Box Warning sits in place:
Suicidal thoughts in younger space.
So monitor mood as weeks go on,

Especially when **energy returns** at dawn.

Also risk for **QT prolong**,

Especially when the dose is strong.

Over **40 mg**? Nope, we chill—

Too risky for that **cardiac thrill**.

Serotonin syndrome is real,

If **tripled up** with the wrong meal—

Like **MAOIs**, **tramadol**, or **St. John's tea**,

Can cause **confusion, tremor, fever spree**.

Teach: **No sudden stop**, taper slow,

Or **discontinuation symptoms** grow.

Take with food if GI's upset,

And tell them that they shouldn't fret—

If it takes time, that's normal here,

This med moves slow, not disappear.

Avoid **alcohol**, rise up wise,

And **report if suicide thoughts arise**.

Citalopram, mood's gentle tide,

That nurses guide with strength and pride.

With patience, checks, and timing neat,

You'll help this SSRI bring heat.

Clonazepam (Klonopin)

Benzodiazepine – Anxiolytic / Anticonvulsant / Sedative

Clonazepam, long and low,
A **benzo** with that **chill-time flow**.
Used for **seizures**, **panic**, and more,
It opens up the **GABA** door.
It slows the brain when it's too tight,
Brings **anxiolytic** calm and night.
Helps with **panic attacks**, intense and sharp,
And **epilepsy** that won't depart.

Oral tabs, and **ODTs**,
Takes effect quite rapidly.
Long **half-life**? Oh you bet—
This med can linger like a threat.
Side effects? We've seen the scroll:
Drowsiness, dizzy, slow control.
Ataxia, confusion, blurred-out brain,
And **memory loss** if it stays in lane.

Black Box Warning, loud and real:
With **opioids**, it's a deadly deal.

Risk of **respiratory depression** climbs—
So watch those **polypharmacy times**.
Also : **Dependence** risk is high,
Even with folks who "just comply."
So **short-term use** is nurse's aim,
And **taper slowly**—that's the game.

Not for folks with **sleep apnea**,
Or **severe liver damage drama**.
And in older adults, fall risk flies—
So start **low**, and **supervise**.
Teach: **No alcohol, no driving fate**,
This isn't one you medicate late.
Take as prescribed, lock it away,
And **don't mix with meds** that make you sway.

Clonazepam—smooth but deep,
Can calm the brain or steal your sleep.
With **nurse-led checks** and patient grace,
You'll guide this benzo in the right space.

Clonidine (Catapres)

Alpha-2 Adrenergic Agonist – Antihypertensive / ADHD / Withdrawal Aid

Clonidine, calm in a pill,
Brings that **sympathetic surge** to chill.
An **alpha-2 agonist**, works upstream,
Shuts down **norepinephrine's** wild dream.
Used for **hypertension** first in line,
But now it's got a **bigger design**:
ADHD, opioid withdrawal, too,
And **anxiety spikes** it can subdue.

PO tabs, patches (wear them slow),
Weekly patch change, clean and low.
Apply to **hairless, rotated skin**,
Fold it after removal—bin.
Side effects? You'll want to track:
Dry mouth, sedation, BP crack.
Bradycardia and **fatigue** may rise,
And **rebound hypertension** if dosing flies.

No Black Box Warning, but hear this bell:

Do NOT stop suddenly, or BP swells.

Taper slow to keep things safe,

Or they'll crash out in a hypertensive chafe.

In **peds with ADHD**, watch their pace—

It **calms impulsive minds** with grace.

Given at **night** to knock out stress,

But **sedation** still may cause a mess.

Teach: Don't mix with **alcohol games**,

And watch for **dizzy, vision flames**.

Tell them to **rise slow**, hydrate well,

And **rotate patch sites** so skin won't yell.

Clonidine—the quiet force,

Slows the nervous system's course.

With **nurse support** and guided hand,

This med can really help them stand.

Clozapine (Clozaril)

Atypical Antipsychotic – Dopamine & Serotonin Antagonist

Clozapine, the final call,
For when **psychosis** breaks the wall.
Reserved for **treatment-resistant minds**,
When nothing else can break the binds.
It blocks **dopamine** strong and wide,
But also keeps **serotonin** in stride.
Helps with **negative symptoms**, too—
Like **flat affect**, or **mood that's blue**.

But this one's got a **dangerous twist**,
So nurses gotta know the list:
It causes **agranulocytosis**,
That's **WBCs dropping like locusts**.
Black Box Warnings? Not one—there's five:
Let's run them down to keep folks alive:
Agranulocytosis — infection risk high
    1. **Seizures** — dose-dependent, no lie
    2. **Myocarditis / Cardiomyopathy**
    3. **Orthostatic hypotension / collapse, possibly fatal**
    4. **Increased mortality in elderly psychosis**

CLOZAPINE (CLOZARIL)

Yup. This one's a **monitoring beast**.

ANC labs are required strict—

No script without that **bloodwork ticked**.

Baseline must be **1,500+**,

Then **weekly labs** for safety trust.

Side effects? Oh, you'll see:

Sedation, drooling, tachycardy.

Weight gain, lipids, diabetes, rise—

It hits that **metabolic prize**.

Teach: Don't stop it on a whim,

Or **psychotic relapse** gets grim.

If **ANC drops**, you'll pause the plan—

And alert the doc as fast as you can.

No **benzos together on first dose day**,

Risk of **collapse** could come their way.

And **smoking** reduces levels fast—

So changes in habits? Flag that blast.

Clozapine—the big red line,

Requires a nurse who reads every sign.

With **lab checks**, **teaching**, and strict review,

You'll give this med like only pros do.

Clorazepate (Tranxene)

Benzodiazepine – Anxiolytic / Anticonvulsant / Sedative

Clorazepate, long-acting smooth,
A **benzo** built to **chill and soothe**.
Used for **anxiety's racing fire**,
And **alcohol withdrawal** wired.
Also helps with **seizure tone**,
But it's converted in the **liver zone**.
It turns into **nordiazepam**,
A **diazepam cousin**—yup, that's the jam.

Oral tablet, works real clean,
But may take time to **fully be seen**.
It **accumulates**, so dose with care,
Especially in those who're **older** or **bare**.
Side effects? Like all the crew:
Sedation, **confusion**, dizzy, too.
Slurred speech, **falls**, and **ataxia** walk,
So **fall precautions** are part of the talk.

Black Box Warning rides the line:
Resp depression when **opioids** combine.

So teach them clear: **No mixing games**,
Or breathing loss might stake its claims.
Also risk for **dependency**,
Tolerance, withdrawal, potential spree.
So **short-term use** is always best,
And **taper slow** if they want to rest.

In **alcohol detox**, it's got its place,
Controls **seizures** and **agitated space**.
But monitor **vitals, neuro signs**,
And dose with care, not reckless lines.
Teach: **No alcohol, no heavy machines**,
And watch for **mood swings**, vivid dreams.
Lock it up, and take as told,
This med's not one for loose control.

Clorazepate—smooth and slow,
Needs a **nurse who's sharp to show**
The signs, the risks, the steady plan—
And guide this benzo like a **pro nurse can**.

Desvenlafaxine (Pristiq)

SNRI – Serotonin-Norepinephrine Reuptake Inhibitor

Desvenlafaxine, mood rewire,
An **SNRI** with **norepinephrine fire**.
Built to treat **major depressive spell**,
And push those dark thoughts back in the well.
It blocks the **reuptake** clean and tight,
Of **serotonin** and **NE** flight.
More **energy**, less **crying days**,
That's how it helps refocus ways.

Oral tablets, once a day,
Take **with or without food** your way.
It comes in **extended-release**,
So **don't crush** it — or peace will cease.
Side effects that may show:
Nausea, dizzy, BP grow.
Insomnia, sweating, dry mouth pain,
And **sexual dysfunction** in the lane.

Black Box Warning, loud and clear:
Suicidal thoughts may draw near.

Especially in **youth**, **teens**, and the start,
So monitor mood with nursing heart.
May raise **blood pressure**, so watch that trend,
Especially when doses **ascend**.
Risk of **serotonin syndrome**, too,
With **MAOIs**, **triptans**, or **St. John's brew**.

Teach: **Don't stop suddenly**, taper slow,
Or **discontinuation symptoms** grow.
Brain zaps, **agitation**, mood may spin—
So let the taper gently begin.
Also warn of **alcohol use**,
Can **enhance sedation** or cut loose.
And **no crushing** — let the XR ride,
It's built to **release the dose with pride**.

Desvenlafaxine, smooth and lean,
For **depression** caught between.
With **nurse-led care** and steady tone,
You'll help them heal and hold their own.

Desipramine (Norpramin)

Tricyclic Antidepressant (TCA) – Norepinephrine Reuptake Inhibitor

Desipramine, TCA light,

With **less sedation**, but still fights the fight.

It hits **norepinephrine** with clean intent,

For **depression** that's tough and deeply spent.

Used in **MDD** that won't let go,

And **off-label** for **ADHD flow**.

Also sometimes used for **nerve pain's sting**,

But it's that mood boost it loves to bring.

It's **less anticholinergic**, which is rare,

For a TCA, it's kinda fair.

Still—don't get too cozy, friend—

'Cause **side effects** will still descend.

We're talkin' **dry mouth**, **constipation**,

Dizzy, **blurred vision**, and sedation.

But compared to **amitriptyline**,

It's cleaner, smoother, more serene.

Black Box Warning, TCA style:
Suicidal thoughts in **youthful mile**.

So nurses watch for mood that dips,

Especially in the first few sips.

Cardiotoxicity is real,

A **TCA overdose** is no big deal—

It's a **code**. With **wide QRS**,

And fatal outcomes nonetheless.

ECG check before you start,

Especially with a fragile heart.

No-go for **MI history**,

Or **arrhythmia mystery**.

Teach: Take it **daily**, same old time,

And **bedtime dosing** often aligns.

Taper slow, don't just stop,

Or **withdrawal effects** could drop.

Also avoid the **sun's bright kiss**,

Photosensitivity is on the list.

And **no alcohol**, it dulls the brain—

Stacked sedation, CNS strain.

Desipramine, the norepi spark,

For **foggy moods** and **mental dark**.

With **nurse support** and cautious check,

You'll guide this TCA to full effect.

Dextroamphetamine (Dexedrine, ProCentra, Zenzedi)

CNS Stimulant – ADHD / Narcolepsy / Off-Label Depression Adjunct

Dextroamphetamine, mind on fire,
Boosts the brain, builds focus higher.
A **central nervous system stim**,
That helps the **ADHD brain** win.
Also treats **narcolepsy doze**,
And off-label where **depression slows**.
It increases **dopamine, norepinephrine**,
Wakes up the brain and gets it steppin'.
Oral tabs or **extended caps**,
Given **once or twice**—watch the gaps.
First thing in the morning, best to do,
Or **insomnia** might come through.
Side effects? Yup, here's the scroll:
Insomnia, dry mouth, loss of control.
Tachycardia, elevated BP,
And **decreased appetite** routinely.

Can also bring **irritability**,

And **tics** in kids with sensitivity.
Growth suppression is rare but real,
So check those **height and weight** with zeal.
Black Box Warning stamped in red:
Abuse potential—use with head.
Can cause **dependency**, **misuse**, crash,
Especially if they take it rash.
Avoid in those with **heart disease**,
Glaucoma, anxiety, or **manic breeze**.
And always screen for **substance risk**,
Before this med joins the mix.
Teach: Take it **exactly as prescribed**,
And never share—**controlled meds** vibe.
No crushing XR, let it ride,
Or you'll get a **dangerous dose inside**.
Also warn of the **crash and burn**,
When it wears off, mood may turn.
So **plan routines**, **hydration**, food—
To help the brain maintain its mood.
Dextroamphetamine—fast and bright,
But needs **nurse-guided** timing right.
With structure, checks, and honest guide,
You'll help this stim be safe with pride.

Dexmethylphenidate (Focalin, Focalin XR)

CNS Stimulant – ADHD Treatment / Schedule II Controlled

Dexmethylphenidate, focused flame,
A **refined stimulant** in the ADHD game.
It's the **D-isomer** of Ritalin's might,
For **attention and focus**, it hits just right.
Used for **ADHD in kids and adults**,
To sharpen the brain and reduce the jolts.
Also helps with **impulse control**,
And **school, work, task completion goals**.
Oral tabs or **XR release**,
Short or long, your pick for peace.
Morning dosing works the best,
Late-day use? Forget that rest.
Side effects—yup, stims still hit:
Insomnia, headache, dry mouth, grit.
Decreased appetite, weight may slide,
And **irritability** may coincide.

Tachycardia, BP may rise,

So monitor vitals—watch those highs.

And for **youth**, track **growth each year**,

To catch any drop in height that's clear.

Black Box Warning says it plain:

Abuse and dependency stake their claim.

So count the tabs, lock up tight,

And screen for **substance risk** just right.

Contra in **cardiac disease**,

Glaucoma, anxiety, or **seizure breeze**.

And **MAOIs within 14 days**?

Hard no. That's a hypertensive blaze.

Teach: Take it whole—don't split the XR,

Or the release might go too far.

No **alcohol**, and **space caffeine**,

Or side effects could get too mean.

Also warn about the **crash and dip**,

As the dose wears off—**mood may flip**.

So routines, breaks, and sleep on time,

Keep that stimulant rhythm in line.

Dexmethylphenidate, laser beam,

For focus, clarity, and team esteem.

With **nurse support** and structure tight,

This med can help them do it right.

Diazepam (Valium)

Benzodiazepine – Anxiolytic / Anticonvulsant / Muscle Relaxant

Diazepam, the OG chill,
Long-acting benzo, calming skill.
Used for **anxiety**, **alcohol woe**,
And **seizures** when they start to show.
Helps with **muscle spasms**, tension tight,
And in **procedures**, it dims the light.
Also given for **status epilepticus**,
When seizures hit and won't dismiss.

Oral, **IM**, **IV**, or **rectal gel**,
It comes in forms that work real well.
But be aware: it works **real fast**,
So monitor when dosing's passed.
Side effects? You'll feel the flow:
Drowsiness, dizzy, slow to go.
Ataxia, **blurred vision**, **confusion** spin,
Especially in **older adults** within.

Black Box Warning, loud and true:

Respiratory depression when mixed with a few—
Like **opioids**, **alcohol**, or other meds
That slow the **CNS** in sleepy threads.
It's also got that **addictive core**,
So use short-term, not forevermore.
Taper slow, don't ever quit fast,
Or **withdrawal seizures** may come last.

Long half-life—it sticks around,
So watch for **toxicity** that builds up in the background.
Especially in **hepatic disease**,
Go low and slow to keep the peace.
Teach: **No booze**, no driving games,
This med sedates, no power gains.
Take **as prescribed**, and know the signs
Of **OD**, or when mood declines.

Diazepam, the benzo base,
That brings the **overactive brain** to grace.
With **nurse support**, close watch, and care,
You'll use this med with skill and flair.

Diphenhydramine (Benadryl)

First-Generation Antihistamine – H1 Receptor Blocker / Anticholinergic

Diphenhydramine, Benadryl name,
For **itching**, **allergies**, and **sneezy game**.
Blocks **H1 receptors**, antihistamine star,
But hits the brain, so watch the car
Used for **allergic reactions**, swell and hive,
Also helps with **insomnia's dive**.
Treats **motion sickness**, **cough**, and more—
And counters **EPS** from antipsych war.

Oral, **IM**, or **IV drip**,
Fast relief in a single sip.
But watch that **sedation** come in hot,
It's a **knock-you-out antihistamine shot**.
Side effects are what you'd think:
Dry mouth, blurred vision, urine on the brink.
Drowsy, **dizzy**, **constipation** dance,
And **photosensitivity**—sun's not a chance.

No **Black Box Warning**, but don't get cocky—

It's got **anticholinergic** risk, and it's rocky.

Avoid in **glaucoma**, **BPH**, and **elder fall**,

And don't stack with **alcohol** at all.

Teach: No **driving**, no late-night text,

This med could hit you harder than you expect.

Also avoid with **MAOIs**,

And don't use long-term—**tolerance flies**.

Fun fact? It's used in **sleepy pills**,

But not the best for long-haul chills.

Use for **short-term nights**, not the year,

Or **cognitive decline** may steer.

Diphenhydramine, common and cheap,

But powerful when it puts you to sleep.

With **nurse-led care** and teaching clear,

You'll guide this med like a pharm pioneer.

Disulfiram (Antabuse)

Alcohol Deterrent – Aldehyde Dehydrogenase Inhibitor

Disulfiram, the no-alcohol sign,
A **deterrent** med to draw the line.
It blocks **aldehyde dehydrogenase**,
So **acetaldehyde** levels blaze.
What does that mean? If you drink?
Your body flips, your vitals sink:
Flushing, nausea, pounding head,
Hypotension, you'll wish you were in bed.
Sweating, chest pain, palpitations,
Vomiting, blurred-out observations.
A full-on **reaction**, 5 to 30 mins,
If alcohol sneaks in—or on the skin.
Used in AUD, that's the goal,
For those who choose a **sober role**.
Not for withdrawal, not for urge—
But a **behavioral boundary surge**.

PO tablet, taken daily,
Usually **at breakfast**—routine, plainly.
And teaching? This part's key to do,

Let's list the **hidden triggers**, too:

No **mouthwash, cough syrup**, sprays

No **aftershave, hand gels**, or **rubbing phase**

Even **cooking wine** or **extracts sweet**

Could bring on symptoms you don't wanna meet.

No Black Box Warning, but don't relax—

This med can cause some **serious attacks**.

Hepatotoxicity is rare but real,

So check **LFTs** before the deal.

Contra in **heart disease, psychosis past**,

And **cognitive impairments** that don't last.

If they **relapse**, wait **12 hours** at least

Before restarting this boundary beast.

Teach: **Carry ID** or a card that shows,

They're on this med in case someone knows.

And let them know the **reaction stays**

For **up to 2 weeks** after the last dose days.

Disulfiram, the hard "NO" med,

That puts the drinking thoughts to bed.

With **nurse-led care**, informed and tough,

You'll guide this med with steady stuff.

Divalproex (Depakote)

Mood Stabilizer / Anticonvulsant – Increases GABA / Sodium Channel Blocker

Divalproex, the calm command,

Helps **mood swings**, **seizures**, take a stand.

Treats **bipolar mania** at its height,

And keeps the brain from sparking fright.

Also blocks those **migraine days**,

And stabilizes neural waves.

Increases **GABA**, slows the show,

And blocks those **sodium channels' flow**.

Oral tabs, **sprinkles**, or **extended release**,

Dosing depends on patient piece.

Take with **food** to calm GI,

Or **nausea**, **vomiting** might fly.

Let's talk **Black Box Warning** scene—

There's THREE, and all of them are mean:

Hepatotoxicity – watch that **ALT/AST**,

Especially in **kids under 2**, it's no jest.

Pancreatitis – sudden, rare, but real,

With **abdominal pain** that won't heal.

Fetal risk – the biggest one:
Neural tube defects when the baby's begun.
Pregnancy Category D, unless there's no other,
You'll use with caution in every mother.

Side effects? Let's count 'em wide:
Weight gain, **tremor**, **hair loss** slide.
Drowsiness, **GI upset**, and mood
Can shift with this powerful food.
Check **platelets** and **CBC**,
Can cause **thrombocytopenia**, you see.
Also risk for **hyperammonemia**,
So monitor if mental fog is media.

Teach: Don't crush the **ER tab**,
And space the dose if GI's drab.
Watch for **signs of liver pain**—
Dark urine, **jaundice**, labs explain.
Divalproex, the steady stone,
Keeps the mood and neurons toned.
With **nurse-led checks**, labs, and care,
You'll manage this med with clinical flair.

Doxepin (Silenor, Sinequan)

Tricyclic Antidepressant (TCA) – Antihistamine / Sedative / Antidepressant

Doxepin, the sleepy flame,

A **TCA** with a drowsy name.

Used for **depression**, **anxiety**, too,

And **chronic insomnia** pulling through.

Also used in **topical cream**,

For **itchy skin** and **histamine dream**.

So whether mind or derm is sore,

Doxepin might be what they explore.

It blocks **reuptake**—NE and 5HT,

But hits **histamine** receptors with glee.

So sedation comes in strong and deep,

Making this one great for **long-term sleep**.

Low dose for sleep, high for mood,

But side effects? Let's review that food:

Dry mouth, constipation, blurred sight,

And **urinary retention** overnight.

Black Box Warning like the rest:

Suicidal thoughts in youth addressed.

So monitor mood in teens and more,

Especially early, when moods may soar.

Also risk of **cardiac blow**—

QT prolongation, ECG show.

Caution in **heart disease** or meds

That also slow the rhythm threads.

Don't mix with **MAOIs inside**,

Or **serotonin syndrome** could ride.

And for the **elder crew**, go low,

To avoid **falls** and **cognitive slow**.

Teach: Take at **bedtime**, rise with care,

No alcohol, and **hydrate air**.

Photosensitivity? Bring the shades.

And watch for **mood** if darkness invades.

Doxepin—the TCA that sleeps,

That **itch relief** and **calming** keeps.

With **nurse support**, wise and tight,

You'll guide this med through day and night.

Duloxetine (Cymbalta)

SNRI – Serotonin-Norepinephrine Reuptake Inhibitor

Duloxetine, strong and sleek,
For when the **pain** and **sadness** peak.
It lifts up mood and cuts through ache—
That's the **SNRI** double-take.
Used for **MDD** and **GAD**,
Also **fibromyalgia** pain all day.
Helps with **diabetic nerve pain** sting,
And **MSK pain** that chronic life brings.

It boosts **serotonin** and **NE**,
For **mental and physical recovery**.
And comes in **delayed-release cap form**,
So don't you crush—that breaks the norm.
Side effects? Let's make a list:
Nausea, dry mouth, dizzy twist.
Fatigue, sweating, insomnia, too—
And **sexual dysfunction** may come through.

Black Box Warning is a must:
Suicidal thoughts in youth we trust

To monitor close in early days,

Especially when energy lifts in waves.

It may raise **BP**, so check that trend,

Especially when doses ascend.

And watch for **serotonin syndrome** signs—

Fever, tremors, hyperreflexive lines.

Taper slow, don't quit it fast—

Discontinuation syndrome hits back.

With **brain zaps**, mood swings, weird dreams,

And flu-like stuff that's worse than it seems.

Teach: Take it whole—**don't open the shell**,

And warn of **drowsy, dizzy** spell.

It may take **2 to 4 weeks** to start,

So stick with it and chart the heart.

Duloxetine, mood + pain repair,

With **nurse support**, structure, and care.

You'll guide this SNRI with power and grace,

And help your patient find their space.

Escitalopram (Lexapro)

SSRI – Selective Serotonin Reuptake Inhibitor

Escitalopram, Lexapro's shine,
Lifts the **low** and calms the mind.
A **selective serotonin boost**,
That helps with mood when joy feels loosed.
Used for **MDD**, the heavy weight,
And **GAD** that won't abate.
Also tried in **OCD**,
And **off-label** in **PTSD**.
Take it **daily**, same time vibe,
And know it takes a bit to jive.
2 to 4 weeks before the shift,
And up to **8** for full mood lift.
Side effects that tend to show:
Nausea, fatigue, and **libido low.**
Dry mouth, dizzy, sometimes **sweats,**
But generally **fewer side effects.**

Black Box Warning, just like the rest:
Suicidal thoughts in youth—monitor best.
Especially early, when energy returns,

But thoughts are dark and sadness burns.

Can cause **serotonin syndrome** heat,

With **fever**, **clonus**, and **tachy beat**.

So don't mix with **MAOIs**,

Or **triptans**, **tramadol**, **St. John's highs**.

Not for abrupt goodbye,

Taper slow, or symptoms fly:

Brain zaps, mood swings, weird despair,

You'll feel it if you're unaware.

Watch for **hyponatremia**, too—

In older folks, that's nothing new.

Check for **falls** and **confusion haze**,

Especially in those with fragile days.

Teach: No **alcohol**, and **take with care**,

Be patient—it takes time to repair.

It's often better tolerated,

Than others that are more sedated.

Escitalopram, clean and cool,

A serotonin-lifting tool.

With **nurse-led checks**, support in place,

You'll help this med work with grace.

Esketamine (Spravato)

NMDA Receptor Antagonist – Fast-Acting Antidepressant (Nasal Spray)

Esketamine, Spravato name,
Ketamine cousin in the depression game.
Used for **TRD** that won't let go,
And **suicidal thoughts** that overflow.
It blocks the **NMDA** brain pathway,
And boosts **glutamate** in a new-wave way.
Works within **hours**, not weeks to wait,
But this ain't a med you self-medicate.

It's a **nasal spray**, but not at home—
Must be used in a **clinic zone**.
Given **twice a week**, then tapered slow,
With **2-hour monitoring** after the show.
Side effects can feel intense:
Dissociation, feeling **spaced or tense**.
Dizziness, sedation, **BP high**,
And **hallucinations** floating by.

Black Box Warning bold and loud:

Sedation, **abuse**, and **suicide cloud**.
It must be part of a REMS-tight plan,
With **certified clinics** and nurse-led scan.
Check **BP before and after spray**,
And monitor for **drift-away**.
They **cannot drive** or go alone,
So have a ride to bring them home.

Used **with oral antidepressants**, too—
It's **adjunct therapy**, not solo crew.
And **not for use in pregnancy lane**,
Fetal harm's a known terrain.
Teach: It works fast, but needs a net,
Of **therapy**, **support**, and **safety vet**.
This med's for patients **who've tried and failed**,
Not a first line — it's second-railed.

Esketamine, bold and new,
For when old treatments won't pull through.
With **nurse-led checks**, structure, and grace,
You'll help this med hold healing space.

Eszopiclone (Lunesta)

Non-Benzodiazepine Hypnotic – Sedative-Hypnotic / Z-Drug

Eszopiclone, Lunesta light,
Helps the sleepless through the night.
Not a benzo, but acts just right—
Binds **GABA** to turn off fright.
Used for **chronic insomnia's grip**,
With **longer half-life** in the script.
Helps with **sleep onset and staying still**,
A first-line pick when sleep's uphill.

Oral tablet, bedtime dose,
Needs **7–8 hours**—not close.
Take it **right before hitting the bed**,
Or you'll get **next-day grog** in your head.
Side effects? Let's make it quick:
Bitter taste is the number one trick.
Also **drowsy**, **dry mouth**, maybe **weird dreams**,
And rare **hallucinations** in the seams.

Complex sleep behaviors rise:

Sleepwalking, **driving**, **eating pies**.
So report if they act while out—
This med may need to **go without**.
No **Black Box**, but still take care:
Addiction risk is kinda rare,
But it's **Schedule IV**, so nurses know,
To monitor for misuse flow.

Not for use with **alcohol drinks**,
Or **CNS depressants**—that combo stinks.
Avoid in **hepatic impairment** strong,
It'll stick around for way too long.
Teach: Take it whole, **don't split or crush**,
And keep your night routine hush.
Don't take if you've gotta rise,
Like working nights or early drives.

Eszopiclone, sleep's clean queen,
For restful nights and dreams serene.
With **nurse-led checks** and safety near,
You'll guide this med with skill and cheer.

Flumazenil (Romazicon)

Benzodiazepine Antagonist – Reversal Agent / Antidote

Flumazenil, the benzo brake,
Reverses sedation for safety's sake.
Used when **benzos** go too far,
Like **overdose** or post-op star.
It **blocks GABA receptors** tight,
And stops that **CNS-dulling light**.
IV push, it works **real quick**,
But can **wear off fast**, so monitor slick.

Used for **benzo reversal**—true,
But **NOT for chronic users**, boo.
Why? Because if they're **benzo-bound**,
You'll send them into **seizure town**.
Side effects? We'll list a few:
Seizures, **nausea**, **panic** brew.
Also **tachycardia**, **agitation**, fear,
And **re-sedation** if levels clear.

Short **half-life**—so keep that drip,
Or **respiratory depression** might slip.

Especially with long-acting meds
Like **diazepam** still in their threads.
Teach: This isn't your casual call—
It's **emergency use** in a monitored hall.
Not for sleep aid reversal chill—
Only when **benzo risk** is real.

Caution in patients with:

- **Seizure disorders**
- **TCA overdose (contraindicated!)**
- **Long-term benzo dependence**

Dose slow and start **real light**,
Titrate gently, watch that fight.
Vitals Q15, eyes on the screen,
Airway ready, **code cart** clean.

Flumazenil, the fast reverse,
For when benzo calm becomes a curse.
With **nurse-led eyes** and crash cart near,
You'll use this med with **skill and fear**.

Flupentixol (Fluanxol, Depixol)

Typical Antipsychotic – Thioxanthene Class / Dopamine D2 Blocker

Flupentixol, off the grid,

A **typical antipsychotic** bid.

Blocks the **D2 receptors** clear,

To calm **delusions**, **voices**, fear.

Used for **schizophrenia's thought decay**,

And sometimes **depression** in a structured way.

The **low-dose oral**? Energizing lift.

The **high-dose IM depot**? Antipsych shift.

Oral tabs for daily plan,

Or **depot shot** for **monthly span**.

Used where **compliance is low**,

This long-acting route lets symptoms go.

Side effects? Let's run that thread:

EPS comes out ahead:

Dystonia, akathisia rush,

Parkinsonism, motor hush.

Also **dry mouth, blurred vision**, haze,

Sedation, and **weight gain phase**.

Long-term risk? You'll need to watch,

For **tardive dyskinesia's** twitchy notch.

No U.S. **Black Box Warning**, true,

But still apply the **antipsych nurse crew**:

Monitor for **NMS** surprise—

Fever, rigidity, mental highs.

Caution with the **QT line**,

Especially in depot over time.

And if given with **antidepressant lanes**,

Watch for **serotonin syndrome** pains.

Teach: Watch for **mood and motor swing**,

Report **muscle cramps** or twitching thing.

Stay consistent with dose and day,

And **don't stop suddenly**, walk away.

Flupentixol, not U.S.-famous,

But in psych practice, still quite heinous.

With **nurse-led eyes**, labs, and plan,

You'll manage this med like only YOU can.

Fluphenazine (Prolixin, Prolixin Decanoate)

Typical Antipsychotic – High Potency / D2 Blocker / Phenothiazine Class

Fluphenazine, first-gen boss,

For **schizophrenia**, chronic loss.

Blocks **dopamine** at **D2 sites**,

To calm the voices, tame the fights.

Given **PO** or **deep IM**,

The **decanoate** shot's a **monthly gem**.

Used when **compliance** starts to slide,

The depot form keeps symptoms tied.

High potency, so what's the trade?

More **EPS** than meds that fade.

We're talkin':

- **Dystonia** (scary tight),
- **Akathisia** (can't sit right),
- **Parkinsonism** (slowed down step),
    - And **tardive dyskinesia**, a twitchy rep.

Sedation is less, but still may show,

Anticholinergic effects come low.

Dry mouth, **blurred vision**, maybe more—
But **EPS** is the real nurse chore.

Black Box Warning like the crew:
Increased death in elderly with psychosis too.
So don't use for **dementia psych**—
That risk is deadly, not just hype.
Also : Risk for **NMS**,
So watch for **rigidity**, **fever**, stress.
Keep **vitals close**, labs in hand,
And hold the dose if things go unplanned.

Teach: **Don't stop suddenly**, that's a must,
Or **rebound psychosis** breaks your trust.
Stay on schedule with **injections spaced**,
And **report all tics** that can't be placed.
Fluphenazine, powerful line,
For **long-term psych** when structure's fine.
With **nurse-led care** and eyes that track,
You'll help this med hold symptoms back.

Fluoxetine (Prozac)

SSRI – Selective Serotonin Reuptake Inhibitor

Fluoxetine, the first SSRI,
Still goin' strong — no lie.
Used for **MDD**, **OCD**, and **panic**,
Even **bulimia** when it's manic.
Helps with **PMDD's hormone flare**,
And **anxiety** stuck in worry's snare.
Boosts the brain's **serotonin stream**,
To lift the fog and spark the dream.
Take it **daily**, usually morn,
To fight that **fatigue**, help folks transform.
But don't expect a mood lift now—
Takes **2 to 4 weeks**, so teach them how.
Side effects you've gotta note:
Nausea, headache, sweaty coat.
Insomnia, dry mouth, anxious feel,
And **sexual dysfunction**—that's real.

Black Box Warning on the chart:
Suicidal thoughts when treatment starts.
Especially in **youth and early teens**,

So **monitor mood** behind the scenes.

Long **half-life**—like **4 to 6 days**,

So **withdrawal symptoms** rarely blaze.

(But still taper slow, just in case,

Especially at a faster pace.)

Watch for **serotonin syndrome** rise:

Agitation, fever, clonus thighs.

Avoid with **MAOIs, St. John's brew**,

And **linezolid** can cause it too.

Not for use in **hepatic woe**,

Use caution if the **liver's slow**.

And for **bipolar**? Use with care—

It can flip the switch to **mania flare**.

Teach: Take it **consistently**, same time zone,

And let them know they're not alone.

It's one of the best in the SSRI line,

With years of research that still shine.

Fluoxetine, the first to rise,

Still holds strong in modern eyes.

With **nurse support**, patient grace,

You'll help this med find healing space.

Flurazepam (Dalmane)

Benzodiazepine – Sedative-Hypnotic / Long-Acting Sleep Aid

Flurazepam, sleep so deep,
But sometimes it's just **too much sleep**.
Used for **insomnia**, that tired fight,
It brings the **GABA** to shut down night.
But here's the deal—**long half-life** lives,
So even next day, **drowsiness gives**.
Hangover sedation, mental haze,
Makes it risky in the **geriatric phase**.

Given **orally**, at **bedtime call**,
It helps with **falling and staying** through it all.
But nurses know, this one can trip—
And make your patient's balance slip.
Side effects? Let's lay it plain:
Dizziness, confusion, memory strain.
Ataxia, next-day foggy brain,
And **falls in elders** are a major pain.

Black Box Warning? Oh yes indeed—

Respiratory depression when opioids feed.

The **benzo + opioid** mix is bad,

So don't stack meds that make breath sad.

Also : **Dependence**, **tolerance**, build quick,

So **short-term use** is the safest pick.

And **withdrawal** can hit with might—

Seizures, **insomnia**, panic fight.

Teach: Take at **bedtime**, not before,

And **no driving**, till you're sure.

Avoid alcohol, CNS depressants too,

Or this med may overdo.

Not great for those who **sleepwalk roam**,

It can worsen those behaviors at home.

And not a go-to in the **elder crowd**,

Too long-lasting, too benzo-loud.

Flurazepam, a sleepy song,

Works—but lingers way too long.

With **nurse-led teaching**, structure bright,

You'll choose safer options for restful night.

Fluvoxamine (Luvox)

SSRI – Selective Serotonin Reuptake Inhibitor / OCD Specialist

Fluvoxamine, Luvox lane,
Not just for sadness, but **OCD's brain**.
It boosts up **serotonin's track**,
To keep **obsessions** from circling back.
Approved for **OCD** in **adult and teen**,
Where thoughts repeat and rituals lean.
Also used in **social phobia** zone,
And **off-label** for depression alone.

Oral tablets, often **at night**,
Start **low and slow**, then raise it right.
It's dosed **BID** when levels climb,
Because of its **shorter half-life time**.
Side effects? The usual scene:
Nausea, insomnia, sexual routine.
Also **sweating, dry mouth**, shaky nerves,
Like other SSRIs on the curves.

Black Box Warning, no surprise:

Suicidal thoughts in youthful eyes.

So **monitor mood**, especially first weeks,

And teach them what to say when darkness speaks.

But here's what makes **Fluvox** stand:

It's the **most intense CYP inhibition** in the land.

It inhibits **CYP1A2 and CYP3A4**,

So watch out for **drug interactions galore**.

(Caffeine, warfarin, benzos, and more!)

Not for use with **MAOIs**,

Or **linezolid**, or **St. John's tea**.

Risk of **serotonin syndrome's** rise,

So watch for **fever, twitch**, and **dilated eyes**.

Teach: Take with **food** if GI's mad,

And warn them if **sleep** or **energy's bad**.

Takes a **few weeks** to feel the light,

So patience is part of healing right.

Fluvoxamine, the OCD tool,

Less trendy, but still clinically cool.

With **nurse support**, careful med guide,

You'll use this SSRI with pride.

Gabapentin (Neurontin)

Anticonvulsant / GABA Analog – Neuropathic Pain / Seizures / Off-Label Psych

Gabapentin, the mystery flame,
Not GABA itself, but close in name.
It mimics calm in the neural line,
But doesn't hit GABA directly — fine.
Used for **partial seizures** as its root,
But really shines in a different suit:
Neuropathic pain, **fibro flares**,
Postherpetic neuralgia scares
Off-label? Oh, it's everywhere:
Anxiety, **bipolar**, **hot flash air**.
And in **alcohol withdrawal** lanes,
It smooths out **tremors**, **mood**, and pains.
Oral tabs, **caps**, or **solution dose**,
Usually **TID**—not once and close.
Take with **food** if stomach's rough,
And titrate slow—this med is tough.

Side effects you'll need to know:
Sedation, dizzy, edema flow.

GABAPENTIN (NEURONTIN)

Weight gain, **fatigue**, and foggy state,
So fall precautions? Yes—don't wait.
Watch for **suicidal thoughts**,
It shares the **antiepileptic plots**.
And **renal dosing** is required here,
When **kidney function** isn't clear.
Teach: **Do not stop it all at once**,
Taper slow, or you'll feel the punch.
Rebound pain, withdrawal rage,
So stepping down is the nursing stage.
May cause **euphoria** in some folks' brains,
Which leads to **misuse**, especially in pain.
So monitor for signs of drift—
Overuse, **hoarding**, or dose shift.
Not a **controlled drug** (in most states yet),
But **abuse potential**? Yeah—it's a threat.
Especially when **opioids ride the track**,
It might enhance the **sedative smack**.
Gabapentin, flexible lane,
From **nerve pain** to **mental strain**.
With **nurse support**, structure, and grace,
You'll guide this med in every case.

Guanfacine (Intuniv, Tenex)

Alpha-2 Adrenergic Agonist – Non-Stimulant ADHD / Antihypertensive

Guanfacine, the calm it brings,
Tames the brain's impulsive swings.
An **alpha-2 agonist** in the zone,
It slows the **norepinephrine tone**.
Originally for **BP drops**,
But now it's used in **ADHD plots**.
Also helps with **tic disorders** tight,
And **PTSD sleep** through the night.

Two forms:
- **Tenex** = short-acting pill
- **Intuniv** = **extended-release** chill

Used **daily**, usually **at night**,
To offset **stimulant crash or fright**.

Side effects? Let's count the cost:
Drowsy, fatigue, attention lost.
Bradycardia, hypotension, too—
So **monitor vitals** like nurses do.

Also causes **dry mouth**, mood may shift,
And **rebound hypertension** if dosing drifts.
So don't stop fast—**taper low**,
Or BP spikes could steal the show.

No **Black Box Warning**, but take care:
With **other sedatives**, beware.
Can worsen **depression**, make it slow,
So screen for mood before you go.
Teach: Take it **at the same time daily**,
Best with **nighttime routines** mainly.
Avoid **alcohol**, heavy machines,
And rise up slow from bed scenes.

Guanfacine, the non-stim peace,
Helps the **hyper brain release**.
With **nurse-led care**, steady and sure,
You'll guide this med with structure pure.

Haloperidol (Haldol)

Typical Antipsychotic – High Potency / D2 Receptor Antagonist

Haloperidol, Haldol hit,
For **psychosis** that just won't quit.
Blocks dopamine at D2 gate,
To calm the brain, de-escalate.
Used in **schizophrenia's flare**,
Severe agitation, ICU scare.
Also used in **Tourette's tics**,
And **acute delirium** nurse-fix quick.
Given **oral, IM,** or **IV**,
And **decanoate** for monthly spree.
The **long-acting shot** holds tight and true—
For patients who **skip their daily due**.
But here's the twist—**EPS risks** soar:
Dystonia, akathisia, more.
Tremors, rigidity, shuffling gate,
And **tardive dyskinesia** if you wait.

Black Box Warning is crystal loud:
Increased death risk in the elderly crowd.

Dementia-related psychosis? No—

This med makes that mortality grow.

Risk of **NMS** is real and rare—

High fever, rigid, altered stare.

BP swings, diaphoresis—

Call the code and halt the thesis.

Also watch that **QT space**,

It can cause **torsades**—heart race trace.

So get a baseline **EKG**,

Especially if other risks you see.

Side effects also include:

Sedation, dry mouth, orthostatic mood.

But **anticholinergic load** is low—

Compared to others, it doesn't show.

Teach: No **alcohol**, and warn the crew,

That **tremors, twitches**, must be true.

Check for **compliance**, labs, and weight,

And dose **real low** for the start-off plate.

Haloperidol, the psych code blade,

Quick to act and nurse-grade made.

With **vital checks** and structured care,

You'll run this med like a psychaire.

Hydroxyzine (Vistaril, Atarax)

Antihistamine – Anxiolytic / Sedative / Antipruritic

Hydroxyzine, calming wave,
Helps with **itching, anxiety, sleep-depraved**.
Blocks **H1 receptors** in the brain,
But it's got that **CNS-sedating** gain.
Used for **anxiety, panic** states,
When **benzo risks** aren't worth the rates.
Also given for **itchy skin**,
Or **nausea** when the stomach spins.

Oral, IM, or **caps that twist**,
Vistaril for psych, **Atarax** for hist.
PRN or scheduled, night or day,
It keeps the restless thoughts at bay.
Side effects—they're pretty tame:
Sedation, dry mouth, drowsy game.
Blurred vision, GI upset,
And **urinary retention**, don't forget.

No **Black Box Warning**, but don't dismiss—
It's still **anticholinergic** in the mix.

So caution in the **elderly crowd**,

Where **falls and confusion** speak real loud.

It's a solid sub for **benzo stress**,

No **addiction**, no CNS mess.

Used in **alcohol withdrawal**, too—

Part of detox nursing crew.

Teach: Take it **before bed** if sleepy's goal,

Or **20–30 mins** before anxious role.

Avoid alcohol, and **no driving soon**,

It may knock them out by afternoon.

Hydroxyzine, non-addict calm,

For anxious minds and skin that qualms.

With **nurse support**, it holds its space,

A quiet med in the mental health race.

Iloperidone (Fanapt)

Atypical Antipsychotic – Dopamine & Serotonin Antagonist

Iloperidone, Fanapt flow,
For **schizophrenia's thought outgrow**.
Blocks **dopamine D2** and **5HT**,
To clear the noise and help them see.
It's not the first we often try,
But helps when others make symptoms fly.
Given **orally**, **twice a day**,
But **titrate slow** or they might sway.

Why slow? Let's break it down:
Orthostatic hypotension takes the crown.
They'll get **dizzy**, **drop**, or even faint,
If you titrate fast without constraint.
QT prolongation lives here too,
So an **EKG** may be in view.
Avoid in folks with **cardiac past**,
Or other meds that make QT last.

Side effects you've gotta name:
Drowsiness, **weight gain**, maybe **lame**.

Dry mouth, **tachy**, **nasal stuff**,

And some may say they've had enough.

Less **EPS** than older crew,

But **akathisia** still breaks through.

Also risk of **prolactin rise**,

So **sexual dysfunction** could surprise.

Black Box Warning on the chart:

Like all antipsychs, there's a part—

Elderly with dementia psychosis? No.

Increased **death risk**, so let that show.

Teach: **Titrate up**, don't skip a beat,

And warn them not to rise too fleet.

Stay **hydrated**, sit then stand,

And call for help when legs unplanned.

Iloperidone, not first in line,

But works when others can't align.

With **nurse support**, patience, and guide,

You'll walk this med by their safe side.

Imipramine (Tofranil)

Tricyclic Antidepressant – Serotonin & Norepinephrine Reuptake Inhibitor

Imipramine, TCA base,
Old-school mood in a modern case.
Blocks **NE** and **serotonin's reuptake**,
To lift depression, calm the ache.
Used in **MDD**, especially rough,
When **SSRIs** aren't strong enough.
Also used in **childhood night wet**,
For **nocturnal enuresis** set.
Oral tablets, take at night,
To sleep through **sedation's** might.
Start low, go slow, give it time—
Relief may take **2–4 weeks to climb**.
Side effects? You'll need to track:
Dry mouth, blurred vision, GI slack.
Constipation, urine delay,
And **orthostatic** drops might sway.

Black Box Warning in bold:
Suicidal thoughts in the young and bold.

Monitor closely when starting med—

Especially when energy wakes the dread.

Risk for **cardiac toxicity**,

That's why **ECGs** earn validity.

Overdose can cause **arrhythmia** blow—

Widened QRS, and heart rate low.

Also caution in:

- **Seizure disorders**
- **BPH**
- **Glaucoma**
    - This med's **anticholinergic** like whoa.

Teach: Take **at night, no alcohol**,

Hydrate, eat fiber, that's protocol.

No abrupt stop, taper slow,

Or **discontinuation symptoms** may show.

Watch for **mood, suicide, EKG**,

And teach them how their days may be.

It's not a quick fix, but for some,

This TCA is how healing's begun.

Imipramine, old but wise,

Still holds truth in modern eyes.

With **nurse-led care** and structured path,

You'll help them find their mental math.

Isocarboxazid (Marplan)

MAOI – Monoamine Oxidase Inhibitor / Antidepressant

Isocarboxazid, MAOI core,
Lifts up mood by **blocking more**.
It stops **monoamine oxidase A and B**,
So **serotonin**, **NE**, and **dopamine** run free.
Used in **depression**, last-resort track,
When **SSRIs** and **TCAs** won't bring them back.
For **atypical depression** that lingers on,
This med kicks in when others are gone.
Oral tab, take **2 to 4 times** a day,
Start **low**, go slow, monitor the way.
Takes **2–4 weeks** to feel the light,
But the risks? They're out of sight.
Black Box Warning front and center:
Suicidal thoughts may still enter.
Especially in **youth**, new starts, or teens—
Monitor closely behind the scenes.
The BIGGEST danger: **Hypertensive crisis** blow,
If taken with **tyramine foods**, you *know*.
 Aged cheese
 Red wine

Cured meats

Fermented treats

These can spike **BP to the sky**,

With **headache**, **sweating**, and maybe die.

Also with:

- **SSRIs, SNRIs, TCAs**
- **Buspirone, tramadol, meperidine, dextromethorphan**
    - Or you'll trigger **serotonin syndrome**—a life-or-death one.

Must **wait 14 days** if switching lane,

Or **washout period** avoids the pain.

Same for **stopping this med**, too—

To avoid a **med interaction stew.**

Side effects? There's a scroll:

Dizziness, dry mouth, weight change role.

Insomnia, tremor, sexual low,

But it's the **crisis risk** that steals the show.

Teach: **Avoid tyramine, check your meds,**

Even **cough syrup** can mess with heads.

Wear a **medical alert**, just in case,

So EMTs won't make a deadly mistake.

Isocarboxazid, rare but strong,

Old-school med that still belongs.

With **nurse-led checks** and structured guide,

You'll walk this MAOI with pride (and wide eyes).

Lamotrigine (Lamictal)

Mood Stabilizer / Anticonvulsant – Sodium Channel Blocker / Glutamate Modulator

Lamotrigine, the mood swing glue,
For **bipolar depression** pulling through.
Also used in **seizure control**,
But in psych, it plays a different role.
It **blocks sodium channels** with care,
And **reduces glutamate** in there.
This calms the nerves, lifts the haze,
And **evens out those depressive days**.

Start **low and slow** — that's the law,
Or you'll trigger a **rash that drops jaws**.
Titrate **gradually**, no sudden jump,
Or **Stevens-Johnson** might start to bump.
Black Box Warning big and loud:
Serious skin reactions in the crowd.
Not just **mild rash**—we mean **burns**,
So stop the med if the redness turns.

Other **side effects** worth the scan:

Dizziness, **drowsy**, **headache** plan.
Blurred vision, tremor, GI flame,
But overall, it's a **well-tolerated game**.
Also rare: **aseptic meningitis**,
And in combo with **valproate**—watch this:
That combo makes **Lamictal levels rise**,
So halve the dose or risks will surprise.

Teach: **Don't skip doses**, stay on pace,
Or you'll have to **restart the titration race**.
Watch for rash, mood shifts, and more—
And check for meds that increase the score.
Also approved in **epilepsy zones**,
But psych world's where it finds homes.
No **weight gain**, no **sedation drag**,
Which makes it a mood-stabilizing flag.

Lamotrigine, the steady climb,
For **bipolar lows** and treatment time.
With **nurse support**, labs, and grace,
You'll use this med in the safest space.

Lemborexant (Dayvigo)

Orexin Receptor Antagonist – Sedative-Hypnotic / Sleep Aid

Lemborexant, sleep's soft glow,
Blocks **orexin**, the brain's "stay awake" flow.
Not a benzo, not a Z—
It lets your body **rest naturally**.
Used for **insomnia**, long or short,
Helps with **sleep onset** and **maintenance support**.
No **knockout punch**, no memory haze,
Just gentle drift through dreaming phase.

Take **PO**, right before bed,
When you're **ready to sleep**, not ahead.
Needs **7+ hours** in your night,
Or next day may not feel right.
Side effects? Let's count the keys:
Somnolence, **headache**, weird **sleep-DVDs**.
May cause **sleep paralysis** or **dreamy states**,
And some report **hallucinate** gates.

No Black Box, but still take care:
Avoid in **narcolepsy**, that's rare.

And **elderly fall risk** can still apply,

So caution if they're frail or spry.

May interact with **CYP3A4 drugs**,

So check for **ketoconazole hugs**,

Clarithromycin, grapefruit, too,

Can raise levels more than they should do.

Not for daytime use or tasks,

Like **driving**, work, or thinking asks.

And **CNS depressants** should be spaced,

To avoid sedation being misplaced.

Lemborexant, new sleep lane,

Without the **addiction** or **hangover pain**.

With **nurse support**, clear teaching style,

You'll make this sleep med safe and worthwhile.

Levomepromazine (Nozinan / Methotrimeprazine)

Typical Antipsychotic – Phenothiazine Class / Sedative / Antiemetic / Adjuvant Analgesic

Levomepromazine, calm and slow,
A **low-potency antipsych** flow.
Used for **schizophrenia, agitation**, fear,
But more in **palliative care** it's near.
It blocks **dopamine**, like old-school meds,
But also hits **histamine**, so it spreads.
Sedation, anti-nausea, pain,
All bundled in this low-potent brain.

Used when **delirium** clouds the scene,
Or **terminal restlessness** turns mean.
Also treats **nausea, vomiting tide**,
In **end-of-life** care, it's bona fide.
Given **oral, IM**, or **IV line**,
It kicks in fast and chills just fine.
Low doses calm, **higher to treat**
Psychosis loud or pain discrete.

Side effects you'll surely see:

Sedation, hypotension, dry mouth spree.

Anticholinergic load is real—

Constipation, blurred vision, that deal.

Risk of **QT prolongation,**

So get that **ECG foundation.**

And just like others in its group,

It brings **EPS** into the loop:

Tremors, rigidity, twitchy face,

And **tardive dyskinesia**—slow its pace.

Watch for **NMS** — it's rare but true,

High fever, stiff, BP askew.

And in elderly patients with **dementia psych,**

There's a risk of **sudden death spike.**

Teach: It's **sedating,** so move with grace,

And keep them safe in sleeping space.

Use in **palliative** is often PRN,

And may replace **multiple meds** with one pen.

Levomepromazine, old and wide,

In **psych** and **comfort care,** it's applied.

With **nurse-led insight,** safety locked,

You'll manage this med like a seasoned doc.

Levomilnacipran (Fetzima)

SNRI – Serotonin-Norepinephrine Reuptake Inhibitor

Levomilnacipran, Fetzima's name,
A newer SNRI in the **MDD game**.
Blocks **reuptake** of **NE more than 5HT**,
So it gives more energy to the gloomy.
Used for **major depression's weight**,
Especially when **fatigue** won't abate.
It **activates** instead of sedates,
So morning dosing? It resonates.

Given **PO**, once a day,
Extended-release, so **don't cut or play**.
Start at **20 mg**, titrate slow,
Max dose is **120**, if they go.
Side effects? Let's run the list:
Nausea, sweating, insomnia mist.
Increased BP, HR climb,
So check those vitals every time.
Also **dry mouth, urinary hold**,
And **constipation**—yup, that's old.
Erectile dysfunction may come through,

Though it's *less* than SSRIs do.

Black Box Warning still applies:
Suicidal thoughts in youthful eyes.
So nurses watch for mood changes swift,
Especially as energy starts to lift.
Don't use with **MAOIs nearby**,
Or **serotonin syndrome** could amplify.
And wait **14 days** between the switch,
Or things could go downhill quick.

Teach: Take it **whole**, same time each day,
And warn them of **BP that may sway**.
It may help **drive**, **motivation**, focus bright,
But **don't mix with caffeine** late at night.
Levomilnacipran, modern boost,
For **depressive lows** that won't reduce.
With **nurse-led checks** and clear guide talk,
You'll walk this SNRI like a psych nurse rock.

Lisdexamfetamine (Vyvanse)

CNS Stimulant

Lisdexamfetamine, Vyvanse flow,
A **prodrug stimulant**, smooth to go.
Converted in the blood to **dextro form**,
For **steady focus**, long and warm.
Used for **ADHD**, first-line vibe,
In **kids and adults** who can't subscribe
To **short-acting meds** that spike and fall—
This one holds from **rise to call**.
Also approved for **binge eating**, too,
To tame compulsions breaking through.
Curb the urge, **control the drive**,
While keeping daytime strength alive.
Take it **once daily**, morning plan,
Oral capsule or **chewable scan**.
Don't take late, or sleep won't land—
Insomnia's got a heavy hand.

Side effects? Let's break it clean:
Decreased appetite, sleepless scene,
Dry mouth, irritability,

And **elevated BP** or **HR spree**.
Also watch for **mood swings**, crash,
Especially when it starts to flash.
May cause **tics** or **worsen anxiety**,
So psych history needs clarity.
Black Box Warning, loud and real:
Abuse and **dependency** may appeal.
It's **Schedule II**, controlled and tight,
So count the pills and dose just right.
Contra in **MAOI users**, no doubt—
14-day washout or danger's about.
Not for those with **severe heart stress**,
Arrhythmias, HTN, or **CVD mess**.
Teach: Take **same time**, lock it down,
And **don't share meds** around the town.
May seem "safe," but hits the brain—
So **monitor growth** and **vitals** again.
Lisdexamfetamine, long-game star,
For **focus, drive**, and goals that are far.
With **nurse-led care**, structure, and plan,
You'll guide this med like only **you** can.

Lithium (Lithobid, Eskalith)

Mood Stabilizer – Bipolar Disorder / Antimanic Agent

Lithium, the mood ring med,
For **bipolar highs** that race ahead.
Used for **mania**, sharp and loud,
And keeps the mood from crashing downcloud.
It **modulates neurotransmission flow**,
Serotonin, **dopamine**—steady and slow.
The exact MOA? Still unclear,
But its **mood-stabilizing** power is near.

Given **orally**, **BID** or **TID**,
Takes about a **week** for peace to be.
Used for **maintenance** and **acute flare**,
But it's **nurse-monitored** with extra care.
Therapeutic range is **0.6–1.2**,
Above **1.5**, the risk comes through.
At **2.0+**, you're in **toxic zone**,
So monitor labs and make it known.

Toxicity signs nurses see:
Tremors, N/V/D, ataxia, confused speech spree.

Slurred words, **EKG shifts**, muscle twitch—

Hold the dose and call real quick.

Labs to monitor:

- **Serum lithium level** (12 hrs post-dose)
- **Renal function (BUN/Cr)**
- **Thyroid panel** (watch for **hypothyroid** fade)
- **Electrolytes**, especially **Na+** parade

Hydration = **safety**, that's the key,

Low **sodium** or **dehydration** = **toxicity**.

So teach to drink and keep salts right—

Not too much water, but enough for the fight.

Black Box Warning includes:

- **Toxicity risk**
- Narrow therapeutic margin
- Close lab monitoring = essential

Side effects (even when safe):

Fine tremor, weight gain, thirst parade,

Polyuria, metallic taste,

GI upset, handshake haste.

Teach: **Consistent sodium intake**, no crash,

Avoid **NSAIDs, ACE inhibitors**, or **thiazide stash**.

They raise lithium levels sneakily—

So check med lists frequently.

Also not safe for **pregnancy ride**—

Category D, especially **first trimester side**.

Can cause **Ebstein's anomaly** in the heart,

So OB planning? Play it smart.

Lithium, the mood line stone,

Holds the swings like a psych throne.

With **nurse-led labs** and structure tight,

You'll guide this med to stable light.

Lorazepam (Ativan)

Benzodiazepine – Anxiolytic / Anticonvulsant / Sedative-Hypnotic

Lorazepam, Ativan name,
A **benzo** with fast-acting flame.
Used for **anxiety**, **seizure storm**,
And **alcohol withdrawal** to keep them warm.
Also used in **pre-op sedate**,
To calm the nerves before the wait.
It binds to **GABA**, slows the spin,
And helps the body breathe again.

Given **oral**, **IV**, or **IM**,
Works within **minutes**, steady gem.
For **status epilepticus**, this is first—
To stop the brain before it bursts.
Side effects? Let's list a few:
Drowsy, **dizzy**, **blurred-out view**.
Ataxia, **weakness**, slowed-down gate,
And risk for **respiratory depression** late.

Black Box Warning you must recite:

Benzos + opioids = deadly night.
Coma, resp arrest, even **death,**
So watch that combo with every breath.
Also : **Dependence risk** is high,
With long-term use, **withdrawal may fly.**
Taper slowly, never stop quick,
Or rebound anxiety could hit thick.

Short half-life, but hits just right,
So dosing through the day or night.
In **liver disease**, it's still okay—
No active metabolites in the way.
Teach: No **alcohol, driving down,**
And keep it locked when not around.
Take **only as prescribed** and **watch for lows,**
In **respiratory rate** and how alertness goes.

Lorazepam, the calming wave,
For crisis moments nurses brave.
With **nurse-led checks,** you'll guide this med,
To bring the calm and clear the head.

Loprazolam (Dormonoct)

Benzodiazepine – Short-Acting Hypnotic / Schedule IV

Loprazolam, bedtime breeze,
A benzo made to bring on Zs.
Used for **short-term insomnia** flight,
To help the restless find their night.
Acts on **GABA**, slows the spin,
Brings **sedation** deep within.
With a **short half-life**, it fades by day,
Less **groggy fog** to get in the way.

Given **PO**, at **bedtime true**,
One dose only, don't renew.
Use for 2-4 weeks at most,
Or **tolerance**, **addiction** starts to coast.
Side effects? The benzo bunch:
Drowsy, dizzy, maybe a punch
Of **confusion**, **falls**, especially old—
So be careful when the body's cold.

No **Black Box Warning**, but still the code:
Don't mix with opioids on the road.

Respiratory depression, coma blend—
The nurse's job is to defend.
Risk of **dependence**, so taper slow,
Don't quit cold—**seizures** might show.
Also **rebound insomnia** may flare,
If they stop fast without nurse care.

Teach: Take at **night**, right before bed,
No alcohol, or sleepy dread.
Lock it up, don't share it out,
And **avoid machines** until there's no doubt.
Loprazolam, the sleep switch flip,
A calm descent, a drowsy dip.
With **nurse-led teaching**, short and clear,
You'll keep this med safe year to year.

Lormetazepam (Noctamid)

Benzodiazepine – Short-Acting Hypnotic / Sedative / Schedule IV

Lormetazepam, soft night kiss,
For **short-term insomnia** you don't want to miss.
A **benzo hypnotic**, fast and light,
Helps patients drift into restful night.
Acts on **GABA-A**, smooths the brain,
Slows the thoughts and eases strain.
With **short onset**, works real quick—
So bedtime dosing does the trick.

Oral tablet, swallowed whole,
Don't crush or split—just play the role.
Start with **low doses**, taper with care,
Or **withdrawal symptoms** may flare.
Side effects? Keep watch and track:
Drowsiness, **amnesia**, attention lack.
Dizziness, **confusion**, **falls at night**,
Especially in **elderly**—watch that height.

Like all benzos, it carries weight:

Dependence, **withdrawal**, tolerance gate.

Only for **short use**, not long-term ride,

Or **addiction risk** starts to slide.

No U.S. **Black Box**, but we still know—

Benzo + opioid = dangerous show.

Respiratory depression, coma, death—

So monitor breathing with every breath.

Teach:

- **Use only as prescribed**, not PRN play
- Avoid **alcohol**, keep sleep routine okay
- **Don't drive or operate** until you're sure
- And lock it up—**diversion's** a blur

Lormetazepam, Europe's sleep spark,

Leaves less fog when morning's dark.

With **nurse support**, clear plan, and grace,

You'll guide this benzo to a safer place.

Lumateperone (Caplyta)

Atypical Antipsychotic – Dopamine/Serotonin Modulator / New-Gen

Lumateperone, smooth and new,
For **schizophrenia** and **bipolar blues**.
It modulates **dopamine D2** tone,
While calming **5HT2A** on its own.
Also hits **glutamate pathways light**,
So symptoms fade and thoughts feel right.
Used for **bipolar depression**, solo flair,
Or with mood stabilizers if they're there.

Oral tablet, once a day,
Take **with food**, keep meals in play.
Needs **350 calories** to be absorbed,
Or the dose might not be fully stored.
Side effects? Fewer, yes—
But still some things to watch and assess:
Drowsiness, dizziness, dry mouth, mild,
And **nausea, sedation** in some filed.

The big win? Less **weight gain blast**,

And **lipids, glucose** tend to last.

Minimal **EPS, akathisia,**

So it's gentler than risperidone's hysteria.

Black Box Warning on board:

Elderly dementia psychosis = death reported.

So **don't use** in that aging crowd,

The mortality risk is still allowed.

Also caution in:
- **Hepatic impairment** (mild okay)
- Avoid in **severe liver failure** way

Teach: Take it **with food**, not empty hands,

And take at the **same time**, per your plans.

Avoid **alcohol**, or CNS may drop,

And if **mood shifts fast**, make a med stop.

Lumateperone, new and wise,

With **gentler weight** and **clearer skies**.

With **nurse-led teaching**, labs, and grace,

You'll guide this med in the safest place.

Lurasidone (Latuda)

Atypical Antipsychotic – Dopamine & Serotonin Antagonist

Lurasidone, Latuda light,
For **bipolar lows** and **schizo fight**.
It blocks **D2** and **5HT2A**,
To clear the fog and hold dismay.
Used for **bipolar depression**, too,
Alone or with a **mood-stabilizing crew**.
Also helps with **schizo flare**,
With **less sedation**, more mental air.

Given **orally**, **once a day**,
Take **with food**, or it won't stay.
Need **350 calories** to digest—
Without that, you won't get the best.
Side effects are mostly light:
Nausea, restless legs at night,
Akathisia, dizzy, mild fatigue,
But not like others in the league.

The **metabolic profile** stays real chill:
No big weight gain, blood sugar still.

Less **lipid rise**, less **prolactin** spike,
That's why docs and patients like.
Black Box Warning in the frame:
Elderly psychosis death is the name.
So no use in **dementia age**,
It ups mortality, flips the page.

Teach: Take **with food**, same time vibe,
And **avoid alcohol** on this ride.
Watch for **mood shifts**, **tremors**, tight,
And teach about **sunlight-sensitivity light**.
Also warn: It may cause sleep,
So caution with machines you keep.
And if they're **pregnant or planning so**,
This med's safety isn't fully known.

Lurasidone, the newer wave,
With **cleaner effects** and brain to save.
With **nurse-led care**, structure, and track,
You'll guide this med and have their back.

Melatonin (Circadin, Slenyto, Syncrodin)

Natural Hormone – Sleep-Wake Cycle Regulator / OTC Supplement

Melatonin, nightfall flow,
Signals the body it's time to slow.
Made in the **pineal gland**, no lie,
It rises when the light says bye.
Used for **insomnia**, mild and light,
Jet lag, **shift work**, **kids at night**.
Also helpful for **autism sleep**,
And calming **ADHD bedtime leaps**.

Over-the-counter, common dose,
But strength and quality can be gross.
Usually **1 to 5 mg** is fine—
Start **low**, then move up line.
Take it **30–60 minutes** pre-snooze,
And dim those lights to set the mood.
No screens or caffeine in the zone,
Or melatonin's work gets overthrown.

Side effects? They're usually rare:
Drowsiness, **vivid dreams**, maybe glare.
Headache, **nausea**, **daytime haze**,
And **mood swings** in a few odd days.
No **Black Box**, but nurses know:
It's **not regulated**—that's the show.
Supplements vary in what they hold,
So stick to brands that test and told.

Teach: Take **same time**, **don't stack high**,
More melatonin won't make you fly.
And it's **not for use with sedatives mix**,
Unless the doc okay'd that fix.
Also avoid in **pregnancy call**,
And teach that it's not for **every fall**.
Used for **rhythm**, not sedation ride—
So it won't knock you out like Z-drugs tried.

Melatonin, gentle night,
For circadian drift and natural light.
With **nurse support**, timing, and guide,
You'll use this aid with skill and pride.

Memantine (Namenda)

NMDA Receptor Antagonist – Alzheimer's Disease / Cognitive Enhancer

Memantine, memory hold,
Slows the brain from growing cold.
For **moderate to severe Alzheimer's days**,
It helps maintain those fading ways.
It blocks the **NMDA receptor gate**,
Stops **glutamate's** excessive fate.
Too much glutamate kills brain cells fast—
Memantine helps those neurons last.

Oral tablet or **XR form**,
Start **low**, go slow, is the norm.
Once or twice daily, food or none,
Adjust for **renal** if need be done.
Used **alone** or **with donepezil**,
To stretch cognition out until
The patient slowly starts to slide—
It gives some time before that tide.

Side effects? They're mostly chill:

Dizzy, confusion, headache spill.

Sometimes **hallucinations, constipation**,

But usually fewer than cholinergic stations.

No **Black Box Warning**, but still take care—

Use caution in **renal impairment** there.

Also watch in folks with **seizure tracks**,

Or **cardiac rhythm** that often cracks.

Teach: This med is **not a cure**,

But helps with **daily tasks** for sure.

Take as prescribed, same time each day,

And report if thoughts go far astray.

Memantine, brain's soft shield,

In memory's war, a gentler field.

With **nurse support**, kind voice, and guide,

You'll help this med stand strong with pride.

Methadone (Dolophine, Methadose)

Opioid Analgesic / OUD Maintenance – Full Mu Opioid Agonist / Schedule II

Methadone, the long-game ride,

For **chronic pain** or **addiction guide**.

A **full opioid agonist**, slow to peak,

But sticks around all through the week.

Used in **opioid use disorder**, plan,

To **prevent withdrawal** and **craving ban**.

Also treats **severe pain** long-term,

But must be dosed with careful concern.

Given **oral tab**, **liquid**, or **dissolve**,

Dosing takes time to **fine-tune and evolve**.

Start low, go slow, watch the build—

This med can **stack** and get you chilled.

Why? Because the **half-life's long**,

Lasts **8 to 59 hours strong**.

But the **pain relief**? Just **4 to 8**,

So dosing errors escalate.

Side effects you'd expect to see:

Sedation, nausea, constipation spree.

Sweating, confusion, QT prolong,
And **respiratory depression** if things go wrong.
Black Box Warning is loud and clear:
Resp arrest, QT risk, so stay near.
Also high **abuse potential**,
So **controlled dispensing** is essential.
Monitor:

- **EKG** (baseline + periodic)
- **Respiratory rate**
- **Mental status**
- **Signs of overdose or withdrawal fate**

Teach: Take **only as prescribed**, no bend,
And **never mix with benzos**, friend.
Avoid **alcohol, sedatives**, too—
Or CNS depression will follow through.
Taper slow if stopping comes,
Or withdrawal symptoms start to drum:
Yawning, sweating, GI pain,
Muscle aches and **moody brain.**
Methadone, complex and deep,
Helps the broken safely sleep.
With **nurse-led structure**, checks in line,
You'll guide this med with skill and spine.

Methylphenidate (Ritalin, Concerta)

CNS Stimulant – ADHD / Narcolepsy / Schedule II

Methylphenidate, focus king,
Brings the brain that **steady zing**.
For **ADHD**, it's first in line—
To help the mind and thoughts align.
Also used for **narcoleptic drag**,
To keep them up without the lag.
Blocks **reuptake** of **dopamine** and **NE**,
So thoughts move with clarity.
Comes in **IR**, **ER**, **XR**, patch too,
So nurses watch the form and cue.
Ritalin short, **Concerta** long,
Daytrana patch for kids that strong.
Side effects you'll need to know:
Decreased appetite, **weight loss show**,
Insomnia, **dry mouth**, jittery tone,
And **tachycardia** thrown alone.
Black Box Warning real loud:
Abuse, **dependency** in the crowd.

It's **Schedule II**, tight and tracked,

So no sharing, hoarding, or script hacked.

Also watch for **BP rise**,

And **growth suppression** in younger size.

Check **height and weight** every while,

And monitor **mood** for darker style.

Teach: Take in **morning**, food or none,

Late doses = **no sleep fun**.

Don't crush XR, don't split the shell,

And teach that **drug holidays** can go well.

Contra in:

- **Tics** or **Tourette's path**
- **Severe anxiety** or panic wrath
- And don't mix with **MAOIs**,
  - Or **hypertensive crisis** flies.

Teach: **No alcohol**, **lock it tight**,

And **follow up visits** keep things right.

Watch for **misuse** signs and slips,

Like craving, doubling, or skipped-out dips.

Methylphenidate, sharp and clear,

A brain boost tool when structure's near.

With **nurse-led care**, vitals, and grace,

You'll guide this med at the perfect pace.

Midazolam (Versed)

Benzodiazepine – Sedative / Hypnotic / Anticonvulsant / Anxiolytic / Schedule IV

Midazolam, Versed fame,
Fastest benzo in the game.
Used for **procedures**, **intubation**, chills,
And **status seizures** needing skills.
Acts on **GABA**, CNS slow,
Brings sedation's calming flow.
IV, IM, buccal, or nose—
It kicks in fast, and really goes.
Given **IV push or continuous drip**,
It's the go-to med when patients flip.
Used in **surgery**, **ICU** sleep,
Or **pre-op nerves** you need to keep.

Side effects you *must* assess:
Respiratory depression—yes.
Hypotension, drowsy, slurred-out speech,
And in the **elderly**, it hits the breach.
Black Box Warning? Not just one:
Resp depression and **cardiac stun**.

Especially if **opioids** join the ride,

That combo could be suicide.

 Also: **Amnesia, paradox react**,

Where the patient freaks and fights right back.

Rare, but real—so nurses know

To titrate slow and watch the show.

Antidote? That's **Flumazenil**,

But use with care or seizures spill.

Especially if they've been on long—

Reversal could go really wrong.

Teach: This med means **constant eyes**,

Vitals, O$_2$, crash cart nearby.

No driving after, no memory near,

And explain the **amnesia** that may appear.

Short **half-life**, but **power packed**,

It's in and out, but you better act.

With **tubed patients** or seizures tight,

Midazolam is nurse-highlight.

Midazolam, the calming blade,

In critical scenes where nerves invade.

With **nurse-led care**, airway checks tight,

You'll guide this med with clinical might.

Mirtazapine (Remeron)

Atypical Antidepressant – Noradrenergic & Specific Serotonergic Antidepressant (NaSSA)

Mirtazapine, Remeron chill,

For **depression** that won't stay still.

Especially when there's **sleep loss**, strain,

Or **appetite gone** down the drain.

It blocks **alpha-2** to raise the game,

Boosts **NE** and **serotonin's name**.

Also blocks **5HT2 and H1**,

So it's **sedating** once it's begun.

Oral tab or **dissolving form**,

Take it **at bedtime**, sleep is born.

Doses start at **15 mg**,

Then titrate slow to find their bang.

Low doses = **sedating ride**,

But **higher doses**? Activating side.

So nurses know: **more is less chill**—

The sedation fades as you raise the pill.

Side effects to watch and weigh:

Sedation, dry mouth, weight gain play.
Increased appetite, dreams, and more,
But fewer **sexual side effects** at its core.
Black Box Warning still applies:
Suicidal thoughts in youthful eyes.
Especially in the starting weeks,
So check in often when the patient speaks.

Teach: Take it **once at night**, same track,
And **don't stop suddenly**, or it bites back.
Taper down with **MD guide**,
Or **withdrawal symptoms** could coincide.
Also caution in:

- **Older adults** (fall risk game)
- **Liver or renal impairment name**
- And **low sodium** risk can grow,
  - So check those labs before they go.

Mirtazapine, the cozy lift,
For **sadness, sleep**, and **eating shift**.
With **nurse support**, insight, and care,
You'll guide this med with calm and flair.

Moclobemide (Aurorix, Manerix)

Reversible MAOI-A – Atypical Antidepressant / Anxiety / Social Phobia

Moclobemide, rare but real,

An **RIMA** with a gentler deal.

It blocks **MAO-A**, but not too tight,

So **serotonin** and **NE** take flight.

Used for **depression**, low and wide,

Especially if **atypical signs** collide.

Also used for **social fear**,

Where panic makes the world unclear.

Reversible, so less concern,

For **tyramine crisis** that makes us churn.

But still avoid that **cheese and wine**,

If doses go above the line.

Oral tab, **BID** or more,

Starts around **150 mg core**.

Titrate up with watchful care,

It takes **2–4 weeks** for full repair.

Side effects? They're usually mild:

Insomnia, **dry mouth**, maybe wild
Nausea, **headache**, **agitation**
But fewer than old MAOI station.
No **Black Box**, but still take care—
Serotonin syndrome lurks out there.
Don't mix with:

- **SSRIs, SNRIs, triptan blend**
- **Meperidine, linezolid**, friend

Avoid if history shows:

- **Bipolar disorder**, mania flows
- **Schizophrenia**, psychosis track
    - It can **worsen mood** and bring symptoms back.

Teach: **No abrupt stop**, taper with grace,
And watch for **mood shifts** taking place.
Take with **food** if tummy's sore,
And dose early to sleep restore.
Moclobemide, the softer lane,
Of **MAOI** power without the pain.
With **nurse support**, global and wise,
You'll guide this med with careful eyes.

Modafinil (Provigil)

Wakefulness-Promoting Agent – CNS Stimulant-Like / Schedule IV

Modafinil, mind awake,

Fights **excess sleep** for focus' sake.

Used for **narcolepsy, sleep apnea**, too,

And **shift work sleep disorder** in the crew.

It's not a **classic stim**, like Adderall's line,

But keeps the brain **alert and fine**.

Mechanism? Still a bit gray,

But likely boosts **dopamine** in a light-play way.

Once daily, taken **early on**,

Or **1 hour pre-shift** if sleep is gone.

Avoid late doses—**insomnia risk**—

Keep that **circadian rhythm brisk**.

Side effects? Usually **mild**,

But here's what nurses may see compiled:

Headache, nausea, nervous feel,

And **anxiety** in some is real.

Rare but serious? It's true—

Steven-Johnson syndrome could debut.

So report any **rash**, even small,

And **stop the drug** before things fall.

May reduce **birth control's flair**,

So **backup contraception** is fair.

And not for use in **pregnancy ride**,

The safety's unclear, so set that guide.

Also caution in:

- **Cardiac issues**, **HTN gate**
- **Psychosis**, **mania**, or anxious state
    - It can worsen mental shifts in flow,
    - So check that **psych history** before you go.

No Black Box, but still controlled—

It's **Schedule IV**, so keep it bold.

Watch for **misuse**, **non-prescribed grabs**,

Especially in students pulling study jabs.

Teach:

- **Take in morning**, or work shift aligned
- **Avoid caffeine stacks**, overstimmed mind
- Report **rash**, **chest pain**, or **mental haze**,
    - And **stay hydrated** on busy days.

Modafinil, the subtle rise,

Keeps sleepy brains sharp and wise.

With **nurse-led checks**, structure, and guide,

You'll use this med with watchful pride.

Naloxone (Narcan)

Opioid Antagonist – Antidote / Emergency Med

Naloxone, reversal gold,
For **opioid overdose**, strong and bold.
Blocks the **mu receptors** clean,
So **respiratory drive** can re-convene.
Used for **heroin, fentanyl, oxycodone's grip**,
When breathing starts to **slow and slip**.
Also stocked for **surgery plans**,
In case the opioids change the scans.

Comes in forms:
- **IV, IM, SC**, or **nose spray** fast,
- **Auto-injectors** for the public cast.
- **Intranasal** for bystander hands—
    - It saves a life where no nurse stands.

Side effects? They mostly stem
From **rapid withdrawal** brought on by them:
Agitation, vomiting, sweating, pain,
And sometimes patients **fight the gain**.

Half-life short — that's a flaw,

So opioids may **rebound in law**.

Keep watching them once they wake—

You might need another **rescue stake**.

Monitor:

- **RR** and **O₂ sat** on point
- **Level of consciousness** at every joint
- Check for **re-narcotization drift**,
    - Where breathing slows after the lift.

No **Black Box Warning**, but don't play—

In a code, this leads the way.

If they're on **opioids long and deep**,

Withdrawal could hit while they still sleep.

Teach:

- **It doesn't replace 911**—just buys time
- **Repeat dosing** may be prime
- Store **in easy access**, not locked away,
    - So anyone can act and save the day.

Naloxone, nurse-world spark,

Brings patients back out of the dark.

With **clear heads**, **fast hands**, and heart in sync,

You'll use this med right on the brink.

Naltrexone (ReVia, Vivitrol)

Opioid Antagonist – AUD & OUD Maintenance / Craving Reducer

Naltrexone, long-term light,

To curb **cravings** and **relapse fight**.

Used in **alcohol use disorder** lane,

And **opioid users** trying to reclaim.

It blocks the **mu receptors** clean,

So **opioids can't activate the scene**.

And in alcohol, though it's not full clear,

It **reduces dopamine reward** that appears

Two forms:

- **ReVia**: oral dose, **daily planned**
- **Vivitrol**: **monthly injection** hand
    - Used **after detox**, not too soon—
    - Or **precipitated withdrawal** hits the room.

Start only after they've been **opioid-free**,

At least **7–10 days** (or longer, you'll see).

If you miss that part, the brain will flip—

Sudden withdrawal = dangerous trip.

Side effects? Let's list them fast:

Nausea, headache, tired blast.

Insomnia, **liver strain**, mood swing feel,
And sometimes pain that's oddly real.
Black Box Warning? Nope, not here,
But still some **nurse red flags** appear:
Monitor **LFTs** before you start,
And recheck if pain hits liver or heart
Watch for:

- **Injection site pain** (Vivitrol style)
- **Depression, suicidal thought profile**
- And if they **overdose on opioids** while blocked,
  - They may take too much — the danger's clocked.

Teach:

- **No opioids allowed**, even scripts
- Watch for **pain meds**, cough syrup slips
- Carry a card that says they're on this med—
  - In case emergency care lies ahead.

Naltrexone, the sober guard,
For **healing journeys** that are hard.
With **nurse support**, trust, and grace,
You'll help them win that inner race.

Nitrazepam (Mogadon)

Benzodiazepine – Long-Acting Sedative / Hypnotic / Anticonvulsant / Schedule IV

Nitrazepam, the knockout spell,

For **insomnia** that won't go well.

It binds to **GABA**, slows the wave,

And sends the sleepless to their cave.

Also used for **seizures**, though rare,

In some pediatric cases with care.

It's a **long half-life** benzo friend,

So **next-day drowsiness** won't end.

Given **orally**, at **bedtime right**,

To help patients fall and stay through night.

But build-up in the **elderly frame**

Can lead to **falls** and **cognitive flame**.

Side effects? You already know:

Drowsiness, confusion, mental slow,

Ataxia, slurred speech, shaky knees—

So nurses prep for these risks with ease.

No **Black Box Warning**, but truth still stands:

Respiratory depression in shaky hands.

Especially if mixed with **opioids**,

Or **alcohol** in dangerous voids.

Also:

- **Dependence, tolerance, withdrawal fear,**
- **Rebound insomnia** if it disappears.
- **Taper slowly**, don't just quit,
  - Or **seizures, tremors**, and rage may hit.

Teach:

- Take **at bedtime**, not before
- Avoid **alcohol**, and **lock the drawer**
- **No driving**, no machines 'til clear
- And use short-term—no full-year

Caution in:

- **Elderly** (fall risk sky-high)
- **Liver disease** (metabolism shy)
- And don't give in **pregnancy**—
  - It's **Category D** for fetal safety.

Nitrazepam, the heavy lift,

For sleep disorders needing a drift.

With **nurse-led care**, timing tight,

You'll guide this med with skill and light.

Nortriptyline (Pamelor)

TCA – Tricyclic Antidepressant / SNRI-Like Action / Anticholinergic

Nortriptyline, TCA zone,
For **depression** that's tough and grown.
Also used when **pain won't fade**,
Or **migraines** start to invade.
It **blocks reuptake** of **NE and 5HT**,
To lift the mood and boost energy.
But it also hits **muscarinic path**,
So **anticholinergic** effects do math.

Oral capsule, once a day,
Usually taken at **bedtime** way.
Start **low and slow**, titrate true,
To keep side effects from breaking through.
Side effects? Classic TCA set:
Dry mouth, blurred vision, sweaty net,
Constipation, urinary delay,
And **orthostatic hypotension** may sway.

Black Box Warning: clear and known—

Suicidal thoughts when youth are grown.

Monitor closely the early weeks,

Especially when energy peaks.

  Also: **Cardiac toxicity** risk,

So avoid in patients with that twist.

Watch for:

- **QT prolongation**
- **Arrhythmias**
- **Widened QRS** if they overdose fas

In overdose: it's no joke—

Can cause **seizures**, **coma**, fatal stroke.

So lock it up and dose with care,

Especially if **SI** is in the air.

Teach:

- Take **at night** for sleepy feel
- **No alcohol**, it breaks the deal
- **Don't stop suddenly**, taper slow
    - Or **withdrawal symptoms** may show

Caution in:

- **BPH, glaucoma, seizure folk**
- And **elderly**—they're no joke
    - Monitor for **falls, confusion haze**,
    - And adjust for age with nursing ways.

Nortriptyline, old but strong,

Still finds its place when things go wrong.

With **nurse-led guidance**, insight, and care,

NORTRIPTYLINE (PAMELOR)

You'll use this TCA with clinical flair.

Olanzapine (Zyprexa)

Atypical Antipsychotic – Dopamine & Serotonin Antagonist

Olanzapine, Zyprexa bold,
For **bipolar highs** and **psychotic cold**.
It blocks **D2** and **5HT2A**,
To keep delusions far away.
Used for:

- **Schizophrenia's** thought storms wide
- **Manic episodes** with grandiose pride
- And off-label use for **agitation control**
    - With **IM injection** to calm the role.

Forms? Oh yes, it's got a list:

PO, ODT, and IM mist.

Also **Zyprexa Relprevv**—long-acting shot,
But that one's got a **monitoring plot**.

Side effects? Get ready, nurse:

This one's got the **metabolic curse**:

Weight gain, lipids, blood sugar blow,
And **diabetes** risk on the go.
Also

- **Sedation** (strong!)
- **Dry mouth, constipation**

- And **orthostatic hypotension**
  - Yeah, you'll see it on admission.

Black Box Warning loud and clear:

Elderly with dementia psychosis = death near.

This ain't for **geriatric confusion**,

Unless you want legal intrusion.

Zyprexa Relprevv (long-acting IM)

Must monitor **3 hours post-inject scene**

Because it can cause **delirium, coma,**

So you need a **certified site**—no diploma, no dose.

EPS? Less than old-school crew,

But still can happen, especially new.

Tardive dyskinesia, akathisia, too,

So watch for **twitches**, pacing view.

Teach:

- **Take at night**, helps that sleep
- Warn of **weight** that starts to creep
- Check **A1C, lipids, BMI,**
  - And monitor **mood** that swings too high

Olanzapine, heavy and strong,

Keeps the mind from drifting wrong.

With **nurse-led care**, labs, and grace,

You'll guide this med in the safest place.

Oxazepam (Serax)

Benzodiazepine – Anxiolytic / Sedative-Hypnotic / Alcohol Withdrawal / Schedule IV

Oxazepam, the slow and smooth,
For **anxiety** and **withdrawal moves**.
A **short-acting benzo**, small but wise,
With **less sedation** and fewer highs.
Used for:

- **Mild to moderate anxiety tone**
- **Alcohol withdrawal** when patients groan
- **Insomnia** tied to racing mind—
    - It chills without the long grind.

It binds to **GABA**, just like fam,
But breaks down through a **simple plan**:
Glucuronidation—clean and neat,
So it's safe for **livers** that skip a beat.
Oral tablets, **TID** or **QID**,
Usually **15 to 30 mg** ride.
It peaks real soft, but works just fine—
A **gentle taper** for the detox line
Side effects? They're pretty chill:

Drowsiness, dizzy, slowed-down will,

But **less hangover** than Diazepam,

Which makes it great for nursing exam.

No Black Box, but here's your list:

Still causes **dependence**, don't dismiss.

Taper slowly, or **withdrawal hits,**

With **tremors, seizures,** and anxious fits.

Teach:

- **Take as prescribed, no doubling up**
- Don't mix with **alcohol** in your cup
- **No driving** till you know your state
- And use **short-term**—don't make it fate

Ideal for:

- **Older adults** with **fall-risk frame**
- **Liver patients** needing calmer game
- **Outpatient detox** with safety net,
    - This is a benzo you won't forget.

Oxazepam, the quiet tool,

Not flashy, but it plays it cool.

With **nurse-led care** and insight bright,

You'll guide this med just right at night.

Oxcarbazepine (Trileptal)

Anticonvulsant – Mood Stabilizer / Sodium Channel Blocker

Oxcarbazepine, Trileptal name,
For **seizures** wild and **moods aflame**.
Used in **partial seizures**, solo or mix,
And off-label for **bipolar mood fix**.
Blocks **voltage-gated sodium gate**,
So neuron fire won't escalate.
It calms the brain's electric thread,
To quiet seizures in the head
Given **PO**, in tabs or **suspension**,
Usually **BID** with dose attention.
Start low and **titrate with care**,
To avoid **side effects** lurking there.
Side effects? Let's roll the reel:
Drowsiness, dizzy, double feel.
Headache, fatigue, and GI swirl,
But the **hyponatremia** is what may unfurl.

It can drop that **sodium low**,
So **check Na+ labs** before they go.
Look for **confusion, cramps, seizure sign**,

Especially in **elderly** over time.

Also rare but serious alerts:

- **Stevens-Johnson** = painful hurts
- **Toxic epidermal necrolysis**, too
    - So report that **rash** if it comes through

Not the same as **Carbamazepine** ride,

But shares that **suicide warning** side.

So monitor **mood**, especially fast—

When treatment starts or dose gets passed.

Drug interactions? **Less than Tegretol**,

But still check if scripts may stall.

Watch **hormonal birth control** track—

It may be **less effective**, so back that back.

Teach:

- Take with or without food,
- Stick to the schedule to keep things good
- Watch for **rash**, **dizzy**, **mental haze**,
    - And come in for labs on scheduled days.

Oxcarbazepine, steady and sleek,

To keep the **brainstorms** calm and meek.

With **nurse support**, teaching, and guide,

You'll walk this med by your patient's side.

Paliperidone (Invega, Invega Sustenna, Invega Trinza)

Atypical Antipsychotic – Dopamine & Serotonin Antagonist

Paliperidone, Invega line,
For **psychosis** that's lost in time.
Used in **schizophrenia**, voices loud,
And **schizoaffective** in the crowd.
It blocks the **D2** and **5HT2A**,
To clear up thoughts and smooth the way.
It's the **active metabolite** of **Risperidone**,
But hits more **steady**, more **long-run tone**.
Given **PO** or **long-acting shot**,
So patients who forget? This hits the spot.

- **Invega Sustenna** = once a month
- **Trinza** lasts for **3-month strength**
- **Hafyera** (new): **6 months long**
    - For patients who need extra strong.

Side effects nurses must scan:
Weight gain, prolactin rise, man!
Gynecomastia, galactorrhea,
Plus **akathisia** could also appear.

Also:

- **QT prolongation** risk is mild
- **Extrapyramidal symptoms** in some filed
- **Sedation**, **dizzy**, and **orthostatic dip**,
  - So teach to rise slow so they don't slip.

Black Box Warning—yep, it's true:

Death risk in elderly with dementia view.

So don't give for **dementia psych**,

That's a contraindicated strike.

Bonus points:

- **Renally excreted**, liver safe
- So **hepatic patients** can still embrace
- But **renal dosing** must be done,
- Check **CrCl** before the run.

Teach:

- **Take PO in the AM** if sedating hit
- **Shake the injection** before you split
- Monitor **weight**, **mood**, **prolactin signs**,
  - And **labs for glucose** over time.

Paliperidone, steady and clear,

Long-acting help for minds that veer.

With **nurse-led checks**, structure, and care,

You'll guide this med with strength and flair.

Paroxetine (Paxil)

SSRI – Selective Serotonin Reuptake Inhibitor / Antidepressant

Paroxetine, Paxil zone,

For **depression, panic,** and **feeling alone.**

Also treats **PTSD, OCD,**

Social anxiety, and **PMDD.**

Blocks **serotonin reuptake clear,**

To boost that mood and calm the fear.

But it's the **shortest half-life** of the bunch—

So withdrawal can pack a punch

Oral tablet, take **once per day,**

Usually in the **AM,** they say.

Start **10–20 mg,** then climb,

But titrate slow — give it time.

Side effects? Oh yes, we see:

Nausea, headache, sexual freeze,

Weight gain, dry mouth, sleepy haze,

And **sweating** in those early days.

Black Box Warning applies:

PAROXETINE (PAXIL)

Suicidal thoughts may arise

In **young adults**, teens most of all,

So nurses screen and monitor calls.

Also known for:

- **Sexual dysfunction** (super high)
- **Anticholinergic effects** (why?)
    - → It's the most **sedating** SSRI
    - → And the most likely to make **dry eyes** cry

BIG red flag: **Discontinuation syndrome**

Comes on **fast** if you zoom the room:

Brain zaps, dizzy, flu-like pain,

Irritability, emotional rain.

So always **taper**, never stop quick—

Nurse-led guidance is the trick.

Not safe in **pregnancy ride**—

Category **D**, with **heart defect side**.

If a patient's expecting? No go—

Safer SSRIs take the show.

Teach:

- Takes **2-4 weeks** to lift the fog
- **No alcohol**, it's not a jog
- **No doubling doses** if one's missed,
    - And **therapy + meds** is the ideal twist.

Paroxetine, strong but bold,

For panic and thoughts that lose control.

With **nurse support**, labs, and guide,

You'll use this SSRI with pride.

Perphenazine (Trilafon)

Typical Antipsychotic – Medium Potency / Phenothiazine Class / Dopamine Antagonist

Perphenazine, Trilafon lane,

For **psychotic breaks** and **thoughts insane**.

Blocks **D2 receptors** in the brain,

To stop the **voices**, **paranoia**, pain.

Used in **schizophrenia** core,

And **severe nausea**—less common chore.

It sits between **strong and mild**,

A **medium-potency** antipsych styled.

Given **PO**, **IM**, or **IV track**,

It starts to calm and bring thoughts back.

Also in **combos** like **Trilafon-Amitriptyline**,

But solo use is where it's seen.

Side effects to track in care:

EPS risks **everywhere**:

- **Dystonia, akathisia** twitch
- **Parkinsonism**—slow-moving glitch
- And **tardive dyskinesia** long-term scene,
    - So monitor **tremors**, face not serene.

Other hits:

Sedation, **dry mouth**, dizzy haze,

Orthostatic BP dips in waves.

And yes, it boosts **prolactin**, too—

So **sexual dysfunction** could debut.

Black Box Warning is known:

Dementia psychosis = **danger zone**.

Increased **stroke and death** reports,

So skip this med in elder cohorts.

Teach:

- Watch for **movement changes**, slow or stiff
- Take with **food** if GI's miffed
- **Hydration**, **fall safety**, rise with care
- And check in if **mood feels rare**

Perphenazine, old-school tone,

For when **second-gens** won't stand alone.

With **nurse-led checks**, support, and grace,

You'll use this med in the safest space.

Phenelzine (Nardil)

MAOI – Monoamine Oxidase Inhibitor / Antidepressant

Phenelzine, Nardil name,
For **atypical depression's** stubborn flame.
It blocks **MAO-A and MAO-B**,
So **NE**, **serotonin**, and **dopamine** run free.
Used when **SSRIs fail the game**,
Or **anxiety + depression** feel the same.
Also helps with **panic flare**,
But it's a med that needs nurse care.

Oral tablet, **TID** flow,
Start **low**, go slow — that's how we go.
Full effects take **weeks to shine**,
But the **risks** are steep by design.
 Biggest danger? You already know:
Hypertensive crisis from **tyramine's glow**.
So **aged cheese**, **wine**, **smoked meat fare**
Are foods you must tell patients to **spare**.

Tyramine-rich foods include:
- **Aged cheese**

- **Red wine**
- **Cured meats**
- **Fermented/soy sauces**
- **Draft beers**
- **Pickled anything**

Side effects can also show:

Dizzy, dry mouth, GI blow,

Insomnia, weight gain, shaky track,

And **sexual dysfunction** may come back.

Black Box Warning clear:

Suicidal thoughts in youth appear.

Monitor **mood**, especially start,

And when energy lifts but pain won't part.

NEVER mix with:

- **SSRIs, SNRIs,** or **TCAs**
- **Buspirone, tramadol, meperidine**—PASS
- Or **serotonin syndrome** could explode,
  - With **sweating, fever,** and **seizure code**

Must wait **14 days** to switch lanes,

Or risk **serotonin syndrome** pains.

Same when stopping — give it space,

Or the crash will hit at a dangerous pace.

Teach:

- Strict **diet, med list check**
- Alert all providers to avoid a wreck
- **Medical ID** is smart and wise,

- For EMTs to recognize

Phenelzine, the last-line gold,

For **treatment-resistant stories told**.

With **nurse-led care**, deep patient trust,

You'll guide this med with skill and must.

Pimozide (Orap)

Typical Antipsychotic – High Potency / Dopamine Antagonist / Tourette's

Pimozide, Orap name,

For **tics** and **delusions** that stake their claim.

Used in **Tourette's**, when other meds fail,

To quiet the **motor** and **vocal hail**.

It blocks **D2 receptors** deep,

To give the brain a calmer sleep.

Also used for **paranoid fix**,

Like **delusional bugs** or crawling tricks.

Oral dosing, start real small,

Titrate slow or **QT may fall**.

Used only when **heart is clear**,

This one brings the **EKG fear**.

Side effects? The EPS show:

Tremors, **rigidity**, **pacing flow**,

Tardive dyskinesia can arrive—

Especially with long-term drive

Black Box Warning in neon flash:

QT prolongation brings a crash.

Can lead to **torsades de pointes**,

So **baseline EKG** is what you want.

Also caution:

- **Electrolyte imbalance** (low K^+ or Mg^{2+})
- Avoid with drugs that do the same thing
  - Like **macrolides, azole antifungals,**
  - Or **antidepressants** that twist the jungle.

Not for:

- **Simple motor tics alone**
- **Children under 12**, not fully grown
  - And def not for **schizo psych**
  - It's **Tourette's-targeted**—that's the mic

Teach:

- Report **muscle stiffness, tongue twitch,**
- Avoid **grapefruit juice** (CYP3A4 glitch)
- Take at **bedtime** if sedating hits,
  - And watch for **heart rhythm** that skips or flits.

Pimozide, the niche control,

For tics that take a deeper toll.

With **nurse support**, structure, and screen,

You'll guide this med like a psych machine.

Prazosin (Minipress)

Alpha-1 Adrenergic Blocker – Antihypertensive / PTSD Nightmares

Prazosin, PTSD light,

To calm the storms that strike at night.

An **alpha-1 blocker**, blood vessels chill,

But its real win? **Nightmares killed**.

Used in:

- **PTSD flashbacks, sleep-time screams**
- And **hypertension**, in old-school schemes
    - But now it's key for **trauma pain**,
    - When sleep won't come, or fear remains.

It blocks the **alpha-1** in the brain,

Reduces **norepinephrine's strain**.

So the **fight-or-flight** goes down at rest,

And patients finally get some zest.

Oral tablet, start off **small**,

Like **1 mg QHS**, that's the call.

Then titrate up **slow and smart**,

Because the BP drop is no light art.

First-dose syncope is real as heck,

So **take it at bedtime**, protect the neck.

And **orthostatic hypotension** wins,

So rise up slow or the room spins.

Side effects to teach and track:

Dizzy, fatigue, fainting back.

Sometimes **palpitations**, mild **headache**,

But most tolerate it for dream's sake.

No **Black Box Warning**, but still—

Use **caution in elderly**, fall risk thrill.

Not typically used solo for BP flair,

But for **nightmares**? It's a breath of air.

Teach:

- Take it **at night**, same time style
- Sit, then stand — rest awhile
- Report **fainting, chest pain**, or fear,
  - And teach that sleep may take a week to clear.

Prazosin, the trauma guide,

For restless minds and pain inside.

With **nurse support**, trust, and grace,

You'll bring this med to a healing place.

Propranolol (Inderal)

Non-Selective Beta Blocker – Antihypertensive / Anti-Anxiety / Antiarrhythmic / Migraine Prophylaxis

Propranolol, steady beat,
Slows the **heart** and **cools the heat**.
Blocks **beta-1** and **beta-2**,
So BP drops and tremors, too.
Used for:

- **Hypertension**, classic lane
- **Arrhythmias** that cause chest strain
- **Migraine prevention**, daily dose
- And **performance anxiety** diagnosis

Also used in **PTSD** flow,
To blunt the **adrenergic afterglow**.
Stops the shakes before the speech,
And keeps that panic out of reach.

PO, IV, and **ER tab**,
Watch for **first-dose** hypotension grab.
Start **low**, go **slow**, titrate the med,
Especially in those with fragile tread.

PROPRANOLOL (INDERAL)

Side effects nurses must scan:

Bradycardia, hypotension plan.

Also **fatigue, cold hands**, depressed feels,

And sometimes **nightmares** in sleep reels.

Don't give in:

- **Asthma**—it blocks **beta-2** in lungs!
- Or **bradycardia**—that heart's already sung
- Or **diabetics** who may miss signs—
  - It **masks hypoglycemia's** warning lines

Black Box Warning:

Taper slow, don't stop real fast—

Or **rebound angina, MI**, won't last.

Teach:

- Take it **with food** if GI upset
- Monitor **HR** and **BP** you get
- Don't crush **ER tabs**—swallow whole
- And rise up slow to keep control

In **psych**, it's that *secret chill*,

Takes **public speaking** down the hill.

1 dose pre-event? Yep, that's the way,

To get through panic without delay.

Propranolol, the crossover king,

From **heart meds** to the **mental health ring**.

With **nurse-led guidance**, insight, and care,

You'll use this med with steady flair.

Pregabalin (Lyrica)

GABA Analog – Anticonvulsant / Neuropathic Pain / Anxiety / Schedule V

Pregabalin, Lyrica lane,

For **nerve pain**, **seizures**, and **anxious brain**.

It mimics **GABA**, calms the wire,

So pain and panic both retire.

Used in:

- **Diabetic neuropathy**, zaps and burn
- **Fibromyalgia**, restless turn
- **Partial seizures**, adjunct track
- And **GAD** to pull stress back.

Binds **voltage calcium gates** in nerve,

To slow transmission, dull the swerve.

Not for GABA direct attack,

But the **CNS slowdown** still comes back.

PO form, **BID** or **TID**,

Dose based on pain and how they cry.

Taper slow when stopping, friend—

Withdrawal risk around the bend.

Side effects? ep, they're there:

Drowsiness, **dizzy**, floaty air.

Weight gain, edema, blurred-out view,
And some get **euphoria**, too.
Controlled — it's **Schedule V,**
Because **dependence** can arrive.
Especially in folks with **addiction past,**
So monitor closely and make it last.
Also watch:

- **Renal function** — dose gets low
- **Angioedema** (rare, but WHOA)
- And combo with **CNS depressants**
    - Can make things sleepy and unpleasant.

Teach:

- Take at **same times**, don't skip fast
- May take **weeks** for full effect to last
- Don't stop cold, must **taper slow,**
    - Or **rebound anxiety** may show.

Pregabalin, for calm and ease,
For **nerves that fire** and **minds that freeze.**
With **nurse-led insight**, trust, and track,
You'll guide this med and have their back.

Protriptyline (Vivactil)

TCA – Tricyclic Antidepressant / Norepinephrine Reuptake Inhibitor

Protriptyline, Vivactil ride,

A **stimulating TCA** on the side.

For **depression, energy drained**,

When others leave the patient strained.

Blocks the **reuptake of NE** bold,

So **mood and focus** start to hold.

Unlike other TCAs that **sedate**,

This one helps you **stay awake**.

Used sometimes in:

- **Depression with fatigue**-type feels
- **Narcolepsy** or off-label deals
- Rarely for **ADHD**, though not first-line,
    - It boosts the **norepinephrine spine**.

Oral tablet, **TID** or split,

Starts low—**15 to 40 mg** hit.

Takes a **few weeks** for mood to rise,

But **side effects** can still surprise.

Common flags:

- **Dry mouth, blurred vision, constipation pain**

- **Urinary retention, heat intolerance** train
- **Tachycardia, BP drop, dizzy rise,**
  - And **appetite loss** in a few surprise

Black Box Warning is true:

Suicidal thoughts in younger crew.

Especially during the starting stage,

So check in often, gauge the gauge

BIGGEST danger = **TCA overdose**

With **cardiotoxicity** that quickly grows.

Widened **QRS**, seizures, coma knock,

So keep that **dose locked up like Fort Knox.**

Teach:

- Take in **morning**, don't delay—
  - Too late and you'll be up all day.
- No **alcohol**, no **double med,**
- And taper slow before it's shed.

Not ideal in:

- **Cardiac history, elderly frame**
- Or those with **BPH** or glaucoma name
  - Check **EKG, vitals**, weight and more—
  - This energizer med keeps score.

Protriptyline, the TCA twist,

For **energy-poor** on the depressed list.

With **nurse support**, structure, and grace,

You'll guide this med in a healing space.

PROTRIPTYLINE (VIVACTIL)

Quetiapine (Seroquel)

Atypical Antipsychotic – Dopamine & Serotonin Antagonist / Mood Stabilizer / Sedative

Quetiapine, Seroquel side,

For **bipolar lows** and **schizophrenic ride**.

Also used for **manic mood**,

And sometimes sleep (though not FDA-approved).

It blocks **D2** and **5HT2A**,

To help keep thoughts from drifting away.

Also hits **H1** and **alpha-1**,

Which makes it **sedating** once it's begun.

Comes in **IR** and **XR pill**,

BID or QHS, nurse knows the drill.

Low doses = **sleep** and calm,

Higher = **mood** and **psychotic balm**.

Side effects? You'll see these fast:

Drowsiness, dizziness, that **sedative blast**.

Orthostatic hypotension, too—

So rise up slow when patients do.

Big one? **Weight gain climb**,

Metabolic syndrome over time.

So monitor:

- **Lipids**
- **A1C**
- **BMI spread**
    - To keep your patient **healthy ahead**.

Also watch for:

- **Dry mouth, constipation vibe**
- **Increased appetite**, sluggish tribe
- And **QT prolongation** may appear,
    - So get that **baseline EKG** clear.

Black Box Warning—you know it's true:

Elderly + dementia = death risk crew.

And like all psych meds with depression tie,

There's risk of **suicide** when lows are high.

EPS risk? It's pretty low,

But **akathisia** may still show.

Less than Haldol, more than none—

So nurses still observe that run.

Teach:

- Take it **with or without food**,
- **Taper slowly** if quitting mood.
- Don't drive until they know their brain,
    - And **report sudden mood** or pain.

Quetiapine, the sleepy shield,

For **thought control** and **mental field**.

With **nurse-led insight**, structure, and guide,
You'll walk this med with skill and pride.

Ramelteon (Rozerem)

Melatonin Receptor Agonist – Sedative-Hypnotic / Non-Controlled Sleep Aid

Ramelteon, Rozerem name,
A sleep med that plays a different game.
It binds to **MT1** and **MT2**,
Melatonin receptors, not GABA glue.
Used for **insomnia**, start-to-sleep,
When counting sheep just doesn't keep.
No help for waking up mid-night,
But helps you drift without a fight.

Oral tablet, bedtime style,
Take **within 30 mins**—sleep in a while.
Works best when **sleep hygiene's right**,
So dim the lights and cut blue light.
Side effects? They're rare and light:
Drowsy, dizzy, maybe night fright.
Sometimes **endocrine weirdness** glows—
Like **decreased testosterone, increased prolactin flows**.

But no **hangover**, no brain fog stew,

And no **withdrawal** when you're through.

That's why it's good for folks who fear

Addiction risk with sleep meds near.

No **Black Box**, no **schedule name**,

But don't mix with **CNS depressants** game.

Also not for **severe liver disease**,

So check those labs before the Zs.

Teach:

- **Take on empty stomach** vibe,
    - Or food may block absorption's tribe.
- **Routine matters** — same bedtime slot,
    - Or this med may not do a lot.

Not for:

- **Sleep maintenance** through the night
- Or when **anxiety** is causing fright
    - But if sleep **won't start** and they're clean-living?
        - **Ramelteon** is what you're giving.

Ramelteon, safe sleep key,

For patients who want dependency-free.

With **nurse-led insight**, rest, and plan,

You'll guide this med with a healing hand.

Risperidone (Risperdal)

Atypical Antipsychotic – Dopamine & Serotonin Antagonist / Mood Stabilizer

Risperidone, steady flame,

For **psychosis**, **rage**, and **mood reclaim**.

Blocks **D2** and **5HT2A**,

To calm the mind and guide the way.

Used for:

- **Schizophrenia** in adults and teens
- **Bipolar mania** in the mood swing scenes
- And **autism-related irritability**,
    - With nurse-led calm and stability.

Oral tab, **liquid**, and **long-acting shot**,

Risperdal Consta lasts the lot.

That's **q2 weeks IM inject**,

For patients who forget or deflect.

Side effects? Let's hit the reel:

Weight gain, **sedation**, sluggish feel.

But biggest watch is **prolactin spike** —

So **gynecomastia** may strike.

Also:

- **EPS risk** creeps up high,

- Especially with **higher doses** nigh.
- Look for **tremors, rigid moves**,
- And **akathisia** pacing grooves.

Black Box Warning for all the crew:

Dementia psychosis = **death risk** too.

So **don't give to elderly with cognitive slide**,

Or mortality risks will rise inside.

Watch for:

- **Orthostatic drops**, dizzy step
- **Metabolic issues**, weight gain rep
- **Hyperglycemia, lipid rise**,
  - So nurses monitor labs and size.

Teach:

- Take at **same time**, food or not
- Don't stop fast if dose is hot
- Report **twitches**, **breast change**, or **mood pain**,
  - And check in if **menses go strange**.

Risperidone, the power tool,

For bringing minds from chaos to cool.

With **nurse support**, labs, and care,

You'll guide this med with clinical flair.

Selegiline (Eldepryl, Zelapar, Emsam)

MAOI-B Inhibitor – Antiparkinson / Antidepressant (Patch)

Selegiline, dopamine rise,

For **Parkinson's tremors**, slow replies.

It blocks **MAO-B**, so **dopamine stays**,

And gives the brain some clearer days.

Used in:

- **Parkinson's** with **Levodopa crew**,
    - To reduce **wearing-off** and breakthrough too.
- And **depression**, with patchy style,
    - **Emsam** patch gives mood a smile.

Low-dose oral? You're mostly fine—

No dietary restrictions cross the line.

But raise the dose? Or use the patch too wide?

Then **MAO-A joins** the ride.

 That means:

Tyramine foods become a threat

Aged cheese, wine, meat = no reset.

Because **hypertensive crisis** risk is real,

So teach your patients every meal.

Side effects to watch and share:

Nausea, dizzy, insomnia flare.

Orthostatic hypotension, true,

Especially in older Parkinson's crew.

Don't mix with:

- **SSRIs, SNRIs,** or **TCA play**
    - Or **serotonin syndrome** may slay.
    - Wait **2 weeks** if switching the track—
    - Or it could cause a **seizure smack**.

Emsam Patch = depression line

Apply to skin — rotate the sign.

6 mg/day? Tyramine safe.

9–12 mg/day? You need that food cave.

Teach:

- Take **early** to avoid the night twitch,
    - Because **insomnia** can flip the switch.
- Don't stop fast — **taper slow**,
    - And monitor mood as they go.

Selegiline, the MAOI blend,

With **dopamine boost** that meds can lend.

With **nurse-led teaching**, trust, and plan,

You'll guide this med with steady hand.

Serdexmethylphenidate / Dexmethylphenidate (Azstarys)

CNS Stimulant

Azstarys, double-name blend,
For **ADHD** that doesn't bend.
It pairs **Serdexmethylphenidate**, prodrug neat,
With **Dexmethylphenidate** for fast-acting heat.
Dex hits quick — **within the hour**,
To boost the brain with focus power.
Serdex breaks down **slow and smooth**,
For all-day calm and attention groove.
Used in **kids 6+**, but rising fast,
For **school-day control** that's built to last.
Take it **once daily**, early vibe,
Capsule PO, or sprinkle tribe.
Side effects? Classic stim:
Decreased appetite, weight goes slim.
Insomnia, dry mouth, tummy ache,
And maybe **mood swings** in its wake.
Black Box Warning is in place:
Abuse, dependency — it's no safe space.

It's **Schedule II**, so lock it tight,

And never **share pills**, that's not right.

Also:

- Watch for **increased BP** and **HR rise**
- Can trigger **mania** or **psychosis surprise**
- Not for **glaucoma**, **tic disorder**, or
    - **Severe anxiety** with racing floor

Teach:

- Take in the **morning** (not at night!)
- Report if **heart races** or **mood feels tight**
- **Growth checks** for kids — monitor well
    - And **avoid caffeine**, as side effects swell.

Don't stop cold — **taper with care**,

Or withdrawal could linger there.

May cause **euphoria** in misuse track,

So nurses keep the **pill count** back.

Azstarys, new but real,

For brains that race and thoughts that peel.

With **nurse-led insight**, structure, and guide,

You'll walk this med right by their side.

Sertraline (Zoloft)

SSRI – Selective Serotonin Reuptake Inhibitor / Antidepressant

Sertraline, Zoloft zone,

For **low moods**, **panic**, and feeling alone.

It blocks the **reuptake of 5HT**,

So **serotonin rises** steadily.

Used in:

- **Major depression**, classic start
- **GAD, OCD**, and **anxious heart**
- **PTSD, PMDD**, panic crew
    - Even kids with **OCD** breakthrough too.

Oral tablet, once a day,

Start at **25–50 mg** and titrate the way.

Takes **2–4 weeks** to lift the haze,

So nurses set realistic phase.

Side effects? Let's break 'em down:

GI upset, nausea town

Dry mouth, insomnia, early frown,

And maybe **sweating** hanging 'round.

Big one? **Sexual side effects** rise:

Low libido, anorgasmia ties.

Weight gain? **Maybe**, though less than some,
Still needs tracking as weeks go on.
Black Box Warning is clear and wide:
Suicidal thoughts may coincide.
Especially in **youth**, early phase,
So monitor closely in those days.
Watch for **serotonin syndrome** pop:
Hyperreflexia, **clonus**, sweating non-stop.
Mixing with **MAOIs**, **triptans**, too?
That's a dangerous cocktail brew.
Teach:

- Take at the **same time** every day
- May cause **GI upset** if taken without tray
- Don't stop fast — **taper slow**,
    - Or **withdrawal symptoms** start to show

Bonus nurse tip:
Safe in pregnancy (Category C),
Often preferred for **perinatal anxiety**.
Monitor **sleep**, **mood**, and **adherence track**,
And follow up when energy's back.
Sertraline, a go-to med,
Lifts the thoughts that feel like lead.
With **nurse-led care**, insight, and grace,
You'll guide this SSRI into the right place.

Suvorexant (Belsomra)

Orexin Receptor Antagonist – Sedative-Hypnotic / Insomnia Treatment

Suvorexant, Belsomra's name,
For **insomnia** that plays no game.
It blocks the **orexin wake-up tracks**,
So sleep can come without the hacks.
Unlike benzos, it won't sedate,
It just tells **wakefulness** to wait.
Used when sleep won't **stay** the night,
To help them drift and hold on tight.

Take it at **bedtime**, but not with food,
Or it may delay the sleepy mood.
Start at **10 mg**, max at **20**,
Lower for elders or if side effects plenty.
Common effects include **weird dreams**,
Daytime drowsy, next-morning themes.
Some may feel **paralyzed** in bed,
Or have hallucinations in their head.

Controlled med? You bet it is.

Schedule IV, like benzo biz.

So watch for **misuse**, though risk is small,

Still teach them not to binge or stall.

Not for narcolepsy's crowd,

Because it may silence brainwaves loud.

And those with **depression** deep or wide

Should be watched with nurse at side.

Suvorexant helps the sleep restore,

When thoughts keep knocking at the door.

With calm nurse guidance, plan, and check,

You'll bring this med its restful effect.

Temazepam (Restoril)

Benzodiazepine – Sedative-Hypnotic / Schedule IV

Temazepam, a nighttime dose,
To help the restless brain decompose.
For **short-term insomnia**, it's used with care,
A **benzo** that sedates the night air.
It binds to **GABA-A**, slows the mind,
Bringing sleep when peace is hard to find.
With a **half-life** that's not too long,
It helps you stay asleep all night strong.

Drowsiness, **confusion**, and **next-day fog**,
Are side effects that may clog the log.
In **older adults**, the fall risk climbs,
So monitor closely during sleepy times.
It's **Schedule IV**, controlled by law,
Can cause **dependence**, and that's a flaw.
Don't mix with **alcohol**, opioids too,
Or **respiratory depression** may come through.

Teach: Take it **only before bed**,
Not during dinner or while thoughts spread.

And never quit cold—**withdrawal is real**,

Rebound insomnia can steal the deal.

Temazepam, a helpful guide,

For patients whose sleep has long denied.

With nurse support and proper plan,

You'll guide this med with a steady hand.

Thiothixene (Navane)

Typical Antipsychotic – High Potency / Dopamine Antagonist

Thiothixene, strong and lean,
For **psychosis** sharp and scenes unseen.
A **first-gen antipsych** in the ring,
That quiets thoughts when chaos swings.
It blocks **D2 receptors** in the brain,
To slow the dopamine-driven train.
Used for **schizophrenia**, voices loud,
Or **paranoia** in the delusional crowd.

It hits fast — it hits hard,
But brings **EPS** as the calling card.
Tremors, rigidity, restless feet,
And **tardive dyskinesia** down the street.
Also watch for the anticholinergic wave:
Dry mouth, blurred vision, constipation grave.
Plus **sedation, orthostatic slide**,
So **fall precautions** walk beside.

No **Black Box** for this specific name,

But it shares the **elderly dementia** game:
Increased death risk in that age group—
So don't add Navane to their soup.
Teach patients to report what's new:
Stiffness, **twitching**, or mood askew.
Sun sensitivity might appear,
So teach them to wear hats out here.

Thiothixene, a powerful frame,
Not often used, but earns its name.
With **nurse-led care**, checks in line,
This old-school med can still align.

Topiramate (Topamax)

Anticonvulsant – Migraine Prevention / Mood Stabilizer / Nerve Pain

Topiramate, the quiet brain,
For seizures, migraines, and mood domain.
A **sodium blocker**, GABA-increase blend,
It calms the nerves from end to end.
Used in:

- **Partial seizures** and tonic-clonic flow
- **Migraine prevention** when triggers grow
- **Bipolar disorder**, off-label track
- And **nerve pain** that keeps coming back

Dosing starts low and climbs with care,
To minimize side effects that may flare.
Taper off slowly if stopping this ride,
Or seizures could swing to the other side.
Common side effects:

- **Paresthesia** (tingles)
- **Weight loss**
- **Cognitive fog** ("Dopamax" nickname's not a loss)
- **Fatigue, dizzy**, slowed-down think—

- So nurses teach what's real, not blink.

Risk for **metabolic acidosis** grows,

So **bicarbonate labs** help track those lows.

It may increase **kidney stone chance**,

So keep them **hydrated** in advance.

Not ideal in pregnancy's path—

May cause **cleft palate** aftermath.

So nurses check and guide with grace,

If family planning's in the race.

Topiramate, a multi-use med,

With careful use, it clears the head.

With nurse support and thoughtful pace,

This brain-calmer finds its place.

Tranylcypromine (Parnate)

MAOI – Monoamine Oxidase Inhibitor / Antidepressant

Tranylcypromine, bold and rare,
For **deep depression** stripped and bare.
A last-line choice when others fall,
It lifts the mood or none at all.
It blocks both **MAO-A** and **MAO-B**,
Letting **dopamine**, **NE**, and **serotonin** run free.
But this freedom comes with rules so tight,
That nurses must guide it day and night.

The danger? **Tyramine-filled meals**,
That spark **hypertensive crisis** wheels.
So aged cheese, smoked meats, red wine—
Are foods we warn to leave behind.
Side effects may also show:
Insomnia, tremor, BP blow.
Orthostatic drops, headaches, too—
With risks that many meds outgrew.

Never mix with SSRIs,
Or serotonin storm may rise.

Give **two-week washout**, taper slow,

Or crisis could begin to grow.

Teach the patient: carry a card,

To warn providers when things get hard.

And track their mood, both high and low—

For **suicide risk** can sometimes show.

Tranylcypromine, the old-school fight,

For patients stuck in shadowed night.

With **nurse-led care**, firm and wise,

This med can help the spirit rise.

Trazodone (Desyrel)

SARI – Serotonin Antagonist and Reuptake Inhibitor / Antidepressant / Sedative

Trazodone, the sleepy side,

Prescribed when thoughts and rest collide.

It lifts the mood at **higher dose**,

But **low-dose** use is sleep's main boast.

It blocks **5HT2** and **reuptakes less**,

So serotonin levels can de-stress.

Also hits **histamine and alpha zones**,

Which makes it heavy in sleep tones.

Used in:

- **Major depressive disorder**, full
- **Insomnia** (off-label, but powerful pull)
- **Anxiety, ICU sleep care**,
    - It's everywhere nurses are aware.

Common side effects include:

- **Sedation, dizziness**, feeling subdued
- **Orthostatic drops**, fall risk rise
- And **dry mouth**, blurring sleepy eyes

Watch for:

- **Priapism** — rare but real
- A **painful erection** that won't repeal
- Teach to report if hours tick
    - Or it could cause long-term stick

No **Black Box Warning** of its own,

But shares the **suicidal tone**

That all antidepressants carry near—

Especially when youth are near.

Take it **at bedtime**, that's the call,

Helps them sleep without the fall.

Start low, go slow, as needed guide—

With **nurse-led structure** right beside.

Trazodone, the soft-night med,

That quiets chaos in the head.

With skillful care and eyes on cue,

You'll help this med do what it's meant to do.

Triazolam (Halcion)

Benzodiazepine – Sedative-Hypnotic / Schedule IV

Triazolam, Halcion's name,
For **sleep-onset** that won't tame.
A **benzo** that hits the brain real quick,
But fades out fast like a magic trick.
Used for **insomnia**, short and tight,
It helps them drift into the night.
But don't expect it to hold them long—
This med is for the **falling-asleep song**.

It binds to **GABA-A**, slows it down,
Quiets the mind, softens the frown.
But with its speed comes risky flare,
So nurses guide with extra care.
Amnesia, rebound, sleep-behavior strange,
Like **sleepwalking** or **memory change**.
And in the elderly, that fall risk climbs—
So nurses double-check dosing times.

Short-term only—not for the haul,
Or tolerance and withdrawal may call.

Don't quit fast or seizures spark—
Taper slow and avoid the dark.
It's **Schedule IV**, controlled and tight,
No doubling doses in the night.
Teach patients: **take at bedtime true**,
And never mix with **alcohol** too.

Triazolam, the fast-acting ride,
For fleeting nights with thoughts too wide.
With nurse-led care and structure keen,
You'll keep this med calm and clean.

Trifluoperazine (Stelazine)

Typical Antipsychotic – High Potency / Phenothiazine Class / Dopamine Antagonist

Trifluoperazine, Stelazine strong,
Blocks **dopamine** when thoughts go wrong.
Used in **schizophrenia's** twisting thread,
And sometimes for **anxious minds** misled.
It's a **first-gen**, high in strength,
With **EPS risks** at arm's length.
Tremors, rigidity, restless pace,
And **tardive signs** in the face.

It's rarely used for **anxiety care**,
But **low-dose** only — nurses beware.
The FDA still backs that claim,
But newer meds now take that lane.
Oral or IM, both are used,
But **daily dosing** must be infused.
No long-acting depot form,
Just scheduled meds to meet the norm.

Side effects may also show:

Sedation, dizzy, movement woe.

And watch the **QT interval,**

It can extend — be critical.

Black Box Warning is no surprise:

Elderly dementia = death risk rise.

So don't prescribe in those who roam

With **memory loss** or **wandering home.**

Teach: Report any **muscle twitch,**

Eye rolling, jaw lock, or mental glitch.

Sunburn risk may also spike,

So **sun protection** is just right.

Trifluoperazine, old-school fire,

Still used when symptoms won't retire.

With nurse support, labs, and guide,

You'll walk this med with cautious pride.

Trimipramine (Surmontil)

Tricyclic Antidepressant – Sedating / Antidepressant

Trimipramine, slow and deep,
For thoughts that ache and steal your sleep.
It lifts the mood with gentle tone,
And helps the restless mind disown.
Unlike the TCAs that wake,
This one helps the body break.
A **sedating force**, soft but firm,
For **depression** running long-term.

It works through **histamine block** and more,
And **serotonin** you can't ignore.
Its **anticholinergic** load is light,
But **orthostatic drops** still come at night.
Given **orally**, once a day,
Often at bedtime — the drowsy way.
Start at **25 mg**, then rise,
While nurses watch for lows and highs.

Side effects may come on slow:
Weight gain, **fatigue**, and **dry mouth** flow.

Dizziness, too, and in some hearts,

QT prolongation may take part.

Teach patients not to stop too fast,

Or **withdrawal symptoms** might just last.

Taper slow, with guidance clear,

And check in when they start to veer.

Trimipramine, a softer med,

For heavy thoughts and anxious dread.

With **nurse-led care**, support, and guide,

You'll help this TCA turn the tide.

Valproate (Depakote, Depakene, Valproic Acid)

Anticonvulsant (Antiepileptic)

Valproate, a stabilizing tide,

For **mood swings**, seizures, storms inside.

Used in **bipolar**, both manic and wild,

And in **epileptic** or **migraine-stuck** child.

It raises **GABA**, slows the flame,

Calms the cortex, tames the game.

A first-line choice for mood control,

But comes with risks nurses patrol.

Watch for:

- **Hepatotoxicity**, especially in youth
- **Pancreatitis**, with sudden truth
- And in **pregnancy**, it's a known harm,
  - Linked to **birth defects**, brain and arm.

Labs are key with this med in tow:

Check **LFTs**, **amylase**, and **platelets** flow.

Also monitor for **drug level range**,

Between **50–100 mcg/mL** to keep it sane.

Side effects: **Weight gain**, **tremor**, **hair loss**, **fatigue**,

GI upset, and **cognitive league**.

Some may get **rash**, or mood may slide,

So check in often, stand beside.

Take it **with food** to help the gut,

And **never crush DR tabs**, no ifs or buts.

Teach about signs that warrant a stop—

Like **abdominal pain** or when thoughts drop.

Valproate, the grounding base,

That helps the chaos slow its pace.

With **nurse-led care**, labs, and guide,

You'll keep this med safe and dignified.

Venlafaxine (Effexor, Effexor XR)

SNRI – Serotonin-Norepinephrine Reuptake Inhibitor / Antidepressant / Anti-Anxiety

An **SNRI** that lifts the mind,
By boosting **serotonin** and **norepinephrine** in kind.
It helps with **depression, anxiety, panic,**
Even **hot flashes** and moods that are manic.
Used in **major depressive disorder** clear,
And **GAD, panic, social fear.**
It boosts motivation, calms the nerves,
And helps reclaim emotional curves.

Side effects can come with speed:
Nausea, dry mouth, and **sweating** indeed.
Insomnia, dizziness, or **BP up,**
Especially with **XR**—so monitor that cup.
Monitor BP, mood, and **suicide signs,**
Especially in **teens** and **younger minds.**
Check for **withdrawal** if it's stopped too fast,
Taper slowly, make the healing last.

Teach the patient: don't skip a day,

Or **discontinuation syndrome** may come their way.

May take **weeks to feel the lift**,

So hold tight while it starts to shift.

Yes—there **is a black box warning** due:

For **suicidal thoughts** in the young crew.

So close support and follow-through,

Will help the med do what it's meant to do.

Drug interactions? Quite a few:

With **MAOIs**, it's fatal too.

And **serotonin syndrome** risk is real,

With **triptans, tramadol**, and others in the deal.

Vilazodone (Viibryd)

SSRI + 5HT1A Partial Agonist – Antidepressant

A **hybrid antidepressant**, clever and new,
It boosts **serotonin** with a second view.
It's an **SSRI** and a **5-HT$_1$A partial friend**,
To lift the mood and help minds mend.
Used for **major depressive disorder**, clear,
To soften **sadness**, **guilt**, or **fear**.
It may help with **energy**, **sleep**, and **drive**,
As the serotonin gears come alive.

Side effects? They may appear:
Nausea, **diarrhea**, or **tremor** near.
Insomnia, **dry mouth**, **restlessness**, too,
And **sexual side effects**—though possibly fewer than a few.
Monitor mood, especially low,
Watch for **suicidal thoughts** that grow.
BP, **weight**, and **GI signs**,
And any behavior crossing lines.

Teach the patient: take with food,
It helps absorption and sets the mood.

Don't stop fast—**taper slow**,

And let them know that **results take time to show**.

Yes—there **is a black box warning**, clear:

For **suicidal thoughts** in youth, be near.

Close **monitoring** in the early phase,

Can help prevent the darkest days.

Drug interactions? Definitely a few:

With **MAOIs, serotonergics**, and **CYP3A4** crew.

Serotonin syndrome is a rare alarm,

But mixed with the wrong meds—it can cause harm.

Vortioxetine (Trintellix)

Multimodal Antidepressant – Serotonin Modulator & Stimulator

A **serotonin modulator**, fine and slick,

It works through **multiple pathways**—not just one trick.

It **blocks reuptake** and **receptors, too**,

To treat **depression** and boost mood through.

Used for **major depressive disorder** clear,

To ease **sadness, fatigue**, and **mental fog** near.

It may also improve **cognition** and speed,

For patients whose focus is also in need.

Side effects? You might find:

Nausea, dizziness, and **dreams that wind**.

Dry mouth, diarrhea, or **itchy skin**,

And rare **hyponatremia** tucked in.

Monitor mood, and check Na⁺,

Watch for **serotonin syndrome**, especially day-to-day.

Also assess for **suicidal ideation**,

In **young adults** or early in medication.

Teach the patient: take with food,

To lower nausea and improve the mood.

Results may take a **week or two**,

So let them know what time will do.

Yes—there **is a black box warning** due,

For **suicidal thoughts** in the younger crew.

So follow up close in the early days,

And screen for changes in risky ways.

Drug interactions? A few to note:

With **MAOIs**, it gets the red coat.

And **CYP2D6 inhibitors** raise the level—

So monitor closely to keep it level

Zaleplon (Sonata)

Sedative-Hypnotic – Non-Benzodiazepine / Short-Term Sleep Aid

A **sleep onset aid**, fast and clean,
For those who struggle with nighttime routine.
Non-benzo hypnotic, short in span,
To help you fall asleep—not hold the plan.
Used for **insomnia**, especially **sleep start**,
But not for **staying asleep** or full-night part.
It's great when sleep just won't begin,
And you need a gentle drift within.

Side effects? Just a few:
Drowsiness, dizziness, and **headache**, too.
Sometimes **weird dreams**, or **memory fog**,
And rare **hallucinations** through the grog.
Monitor sleep behavior, strange or bold—
Like **sleepwalking** or stories told.
Respiratory status in high-risk folks,
And **CNS depression** when mixing strokes.

Teach the patient: take it **right before bed**,

And only if they've got **4+ hours ahead**.

Avoid **alcohol** and **driving tasks**,

And don't crush or chew the tiny masks.

There's **no black box warning**, but still be clear:

It **can be habit-forming** if taken all year.

So **short-term use** is the safer way,

And reevaluate if they stray.

Drug interactions? Yes—beware:

With **CNS depressants**, the risk is there.

Also avoid with **cimetidine**,

It increases levels behind the scene.

Ziprasidone (Geodon)

Atypical Antipsychotic – Dopamine & Serotonin Antagonist

An **atypical antipsychotic** calm,
It treats **mania**, **psychosis**, and keeps things calm.
Blocks dopamine and serotonin, too,
To stabilize thoughts and **mood swings** through.
Used for **schizophrenia**, **bipolar highs**,
And **agitation** when logic flies.
It helps with **hallucinations**, **rage**, and **flare**,
And brings the brain back into care.

Side effects? They're good to know:
Sedation, dizziness, weight gain low.
Akathisia, nausea, QT prolong,
And **restlessness** that may feel wrong.
Monitor ECG before you start—
Especially with **QT risks of the heart**.
Watch for **EPS** and **NMS**—
With **rigid muscles, fever, and distress**.

Teach the patient: take with food,
At least **500 calories** to set the mood.

Don't stop quick—**taper slow**,

And report **palpitations** or if they feel low.

Yes—there **is a black box warning**, true:

For **dementia-related psychosis**, too.

In elderly patients, **stroke risk grows**,

So use with caution, the research shows.

Drug interactions? Definitely some:

With **QT-prolongers**, it can become

A dangerous mix, so check with care—

Like **macrolides**, **quinolones**, and others there.

Zolpidem (Ambien)

Sedative-Hypnotic – Non-Benzodiazepine / Schedule IV

A **non-benzo sleep aid**, short and tight,
It helps with **insomnia** late at night.
Binds the **GABA-A receptors**, chill,
To calm the brain and bring the will.
Used for **sleep onset** or **middle-night wake**,
It eases the mind for **rest's own sake**.
But long-term use may not be wise—
It's for **short durations**, not lifelong tries.

Side effects to monitor soon:
Drowsiness, dizziness, or a **next-day swoon**.
Also **sleepwalking**, or things they do
While asleep with **no memory clue**.
Monitor sleep behavior strange,
Like **driving, eating**, or things that change.
Watch for signs of **depression's weight**,
Or **rebound insomnia** if they stop too late.

Teach the patient: go to bed right after,
Take the pill with no delay or laughter.

Don't take with food, it slows it down,

And **avoid alcohol** if sleep's your crown.

There **is a black box warning** to share:

For **complex sleep behaviors** that impair—

Like **sleep driving, phone calls, cooking at night**,

All while unaware, without insight.

Drug interactions? Yes, for sure—

With **benzos, opioids**, and **alcohol**, pure.

All increase **sedation risk**,

So review their meds before they brisk

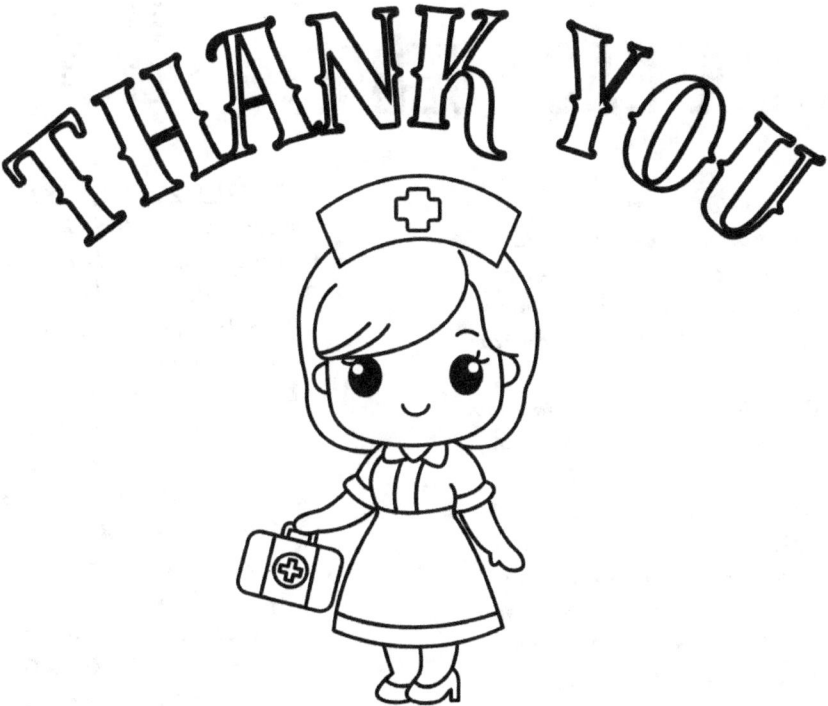

for getting this book and for making it all the way to the end!

Before you go, I wanted to ask you for one small favor. Could you please consider posting a review? Because posting a review is the best and easiest way to support the work of independent authors like me.

Your feedback will help me a ton!

Click **Here** or Scan the QR code below!

OTHER TITLES IN THE MADE EASY SERIES

Pharmacology Series

Geriatrics Made Easy
Emergency Care Made Easy
Critical Care Made Easy
Human Growth & Development
Maternal & Newborn Made Easy
Mental Health Made Easy
Organic Chemistry Made Easy
General Chemistry Made Easy
Pediatrics Made Easy
Med-Surg Made Easy, Vol 1
Med-Surg Made Easy, Vol 2
Microbiology Made Easy
Nursing Skills & Procedures
Pathophysiology Made Easy
Nursing Assessment Made Easy
Nutrition Made Easy
Anatomy & Physiology Vol 1
Anatomy & Physiology Vol 2

Pharmacology Made Easy Vol 1
Pharmacology Made Easy Vol 2
Pharmacology Made Easy Vol 3
Oncology Meds Made Easy
Cardiac Meds Made Easy
Endocrine Meds Made Easy
Pain Meds Made Easy
GI Meds Made Easy
Respiratory Meds Made Easy
Critical Meds Made Easy
ER/ICU Meds Made Easy
Neuro Meds Made Easy
Psych Meds Made Easy
Pediatric Meds Made Easy
OB/GYN Meds Made Easy

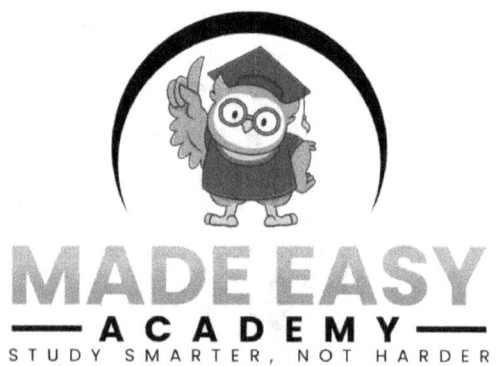

www.ingramcontent.com/pod-product-compliance
Lightning Source LLC
Chambersburg PA
CBHW071020240526
45469CB00006BD/2006